A Radical Guide for ADHD

*Embrace Neurodiversity, Live Boldly, and Break
Through Barriers, Strategies for Conquering
Chaos, Find Focus, and Get More Done and Skills
to Strengthen Executive Functioning*

Alexia F. Randall

Table of contents

Introduction

ADHD stands for attention deficit hyperactivity disorder, a condition with symptoms of inattention, impulsiveness, and hyperactivity. Symptoms vary from person to person. ADHD, or attention deficit disorder, was previously known as ADD. Both children and adults could have ADHD, but signs of childhood still exist.

Hyperactivity deficiency of attention disorder (ADHD) affects children and adolescents and may continue into adulthood. The mental developmental disorder which is most commonly diagnosed is ADHD. Inherently the children with ADHD are hyperactive and unable to control their impulses. And perhaps they have trouble paying attention: these patterns influence the school and home life.

Neurodiversity is a term that recognizes and respects neurological variations like any other human variation. Such variations may include those associated with Dyspraxia, Dyslexia, Dyscalculia, Attention Deficit Hyperactivity Disorder, and Autistic Spectrum. Industry-wide figures can range from 10-20%.

Consider how our brains work; most of us have differences in our tolerance and sensitivities to noise, stimuli, social activity, and how much knowledge we can absorb comfortably until our minds feel overwhelmed and exhausted. We may need to use techniques to adjust to the occupations or environments.

It is very important for us to embrace neurodiversity in every aspect of life. We have to understand the intelligence level of the neurodivergent and help them to grow in it. So, they could enjoy life like every other neurotypical.

There learning producer and techniques should be designed and given to them according to their abilities and talents so they can polish their skills and have a successful career in it.

The neurodiverse people do have to understand their roles as well and should start working smartly so they could play a vital role in society and fulfill their responsibilities and live life fully with appreciation and success.

The women have an important and strong role in our society due to which she has many hundreds of responsibilities to fulfill and challenges to overcome while suffering from ADHD it becomes more difficult for her to get things done.

In that case, she has to embrace her differences, and instead of getting weak or shattered, she has to manage things smartly and get herself organized enough to manage her home with her family and work at the same time. She can use smart techniques, strategies, and use technology to get her things done on time easily and perfect.

Chapter 1: ADHD

ADHD stands for hyperactivity disorder with attention deficit, a disease with signs such as inattention, impulsiveness, and hyperactivity. Symptoms differ from individual to individual. ADHD, or attention deficit disorder, was formerly called ADD. All children and adults may have ADHD, but childhood symptoms still continue.

Disorder of attention deficit hyperactivity (ADHD) affects children and adolescents and may extend into adulthood. The most frequently diagnosed developmental, mental disorder is ADHD. Children with ADHD are inherently hyperactive and unable to control their impulses. Or maybe they have difficulty paying attention: such habits impact school and home life.

For boys, this is more popular than in girls. It is usually discovered during the early years of school when a child starts having trouble paying attention.

Adults with ADHD may have trouble controlling time, planning, setting targets, and holding down a job. They also may have problems with relationships, self-esteem, and addiction. Although it's called adult ADHD, symptoms begin in early childhood and go on into adult life. ADHD is not known or diagnosed in some cases until the individual is an adult. Symptoms of adult ADHD may not be as evident as those of children with ADHD. Hyperactivity may decrease in adults, but it may continue to struggle with impulsiveness, restlessness, and difficulty paying attention.

Adult ADHD diagnosis is close to child ADHD treatment. Care for adult ADHD requires medication, psychological counseling (psychotherapy), and care for any problems of mental health that arise along with ADHD.

Some people with ADHD suffer from fewer symptoms as they age, but some adults still have major symptoms that interfere with their daily function. The main characteristics of ADHD in adults may include difficulties in paying attention, impulsiveness, and restlessness. Symptoms can be mild to severe.

Most people with ADHD are not conscious that they have it — they know only that daily tasks can be a struggle. Adults with ADHD may find focusing and prioritizing hard, leading to missed deadlines and forgotten meetings or social plans. The inability to control impulses can vary from impatience standing in line or traffic driving to mood swings and frustration outbursts.

At some point in their lives, almost everyone has certain symptoms similar to ADHD. If your problems are new or happened only rarely in the past, there is definitely no ADHD in you. ADHD is only treated when symptoms in more than one area of your life are severe enough to cause ongoing problems. It can trace these chronic and debilitating symptoms back to early childhood.

It can be very difficult to diagnose ADHD in adults because certain symptoms of ADHD are similar to those caused by other conditions, such as anxiety or mood disorders. And many people with ADHD also have at least one more disorder of mental health, such as depression or anxiety.

1.1: Types of ADHD

ADHD comes in three types: inattention, hyperactive/impulsive, and the two combined. Males tend to be hyperactive/impulsive in nature, which can cause them to be fidgety, always on the move, interrupting others, becoming anxious, talking a lot, making snap decisions, getting mood swings and being impatient. Females tend to display the inattention type, which makes it difficult to focus, pay attention to details, stay organized, listen, and remember things.

Different types of ADHD, depending on which individual symptom types are the strongest:

·   **Predominantly Inattentional Presentation:** planning or completing a task, paying attention to details, or following instructions or conversations is difficult for the person. The person is easily distracted, or he forgets daily routine information.

·   **Hyperactive-Impulsive Presentation**: The person fidgets a lot and talks a lot. Long sitting still is difficult (e.g., for a meal or while doing homework). Smaller children can constantly run, hop, or climb. The person feels anxious and has an impulse problem. Someone who is impulsive will interrupt others a lot, take things from people, or talk at times that are not necessary. The person has trouble waiting for their turn or listening to directions. A person with impulsivity can experience more accidents and injuries than others.

· Combined presentation: Symptoms of the above two forms are present equally in the patient.

· Because symptoms can change over time, the presentation may also change over time

1.2: Causes and Risk Factors

While ADHD has a strong genetic component — scientists estimate the percentage of the genetic contribution to ADHD at more than 70 percent— it's not guaranteed that ADHD will be passed on to the next generation.

There are several other risk factors for the climate which can play a role. Exposure to certain toxins, such as lead, or certain specific diseases, such as meningitis, may also increase the chances of developing ADHD by an individual.

In addition, poor nutrition or drug use during pregnancy may play a role in developing children with ADHD.

1.3: Understanding ADHD individuals

Here are a reality people with attention deficit hyperactivity disorder (ADHD or ADD) realize from an early age: If you have an ADHD nervous system, you might have been born on a different planet as well.

Many people with ADHD have always understood how different they think. Parents, teachers, colleagues, partners, and friends told them that they did not fit the typical mold and that if they wanted to make something out of themselves, they had better shape up in a hurry.

They were told to assimilate into the dominant culture as if they were refugees, and become like everyone else. Alas, nobody told them how to do this. No one exposed the bigger secret: No matter how hard they tried; it could not be achieved. The only consequence would be a disappointment, compounded by the presumption that they will never excel because, in adulthood, ADHD means they have not tried hard enough or long enough.

It seems strange to term an illness a disease when so many beneficial aspects come along with it. People with a nervous system similar to ADHD tend to be great problem-solvers. They waded into issues that stumped everyone else and leaped to the solution. They're affable, kind people who have a sense of humor. They have what Paul Wender called "relentless determination." They tackle it with one approach after another when they get hooked on a challenge until they master the problem — and they may lose interest wholly when it's no longer a challenge.

I would say being bright, being creative with that intelligence, and being well-liked if I could name the qualities that would assure a person's success in life. I'd choose hardworking and attentive too. I'd like to see many of the characteristics people with ADHD have.

The main obstacle to knowing and treating ADHD has been the unstated and false belief that people with ADHD can and should be like us. For neurotypical and ADHD adults alike, here's a detailed overview of why people with ADHD are doing what they are doing.

Why individuals with ADHD in a binary environment do not work well?

The world of ADHD's is curvilinear. Past, present, and future are never distinct and separate. Everything is right now. Those with ADHD live in a perpetual reality and are unable to learn from the past or look to the future to see the inevitable consequences of their actions. "Acting without thought" is the concept of impulsiveness and one of the reasons people with ADHD have difficulty learning from experience.

It also means people with ADHD aren't successful at ordination— in order to plan and do parts of a job. Neurotypical-world tasks have a beginning, a middle, and an end. Individuals with ADHD do not know where and how to get going because they cannot find the start. They leap into the middle of a mission and, at the same time, work in all directions. The organization becomes an impossible task because it is on linearity, value, and time that organizational systems work.

Why Are People with ADHD Overwhelmed?

People are experiencing life more deeply, more profoundly than neurotypical people in the ADHD community. We have a low threshold for outside sensory experience, as their five senses' day-to-day awareness and their thoughts are always on high volume. Life experiences confuse the ADHD nervous system because its strength is so strong.

The nervous system of ADHD is never in repose. It needs something interesting and challenging to get interested in. Attention is never "deficit." It is always wasteful and is constantly engaged in internal reveries and obligations. If people with ADHD are not in The Zone, in hyper focus, they have four or five things in their heads rattling around, all at once and for no obvious reason, like five people talking to you at the same time. None of this gets sustained indivisible attention. None of this happens well.

Many people with ADHD aren't able to screen sensory input. This is sometimes related to a single sensory realm, such as hearing. The phenomenon is actually called hyperacusis (amplified hearing), even when the disruption originates from another of the five senses. Here are just a few examples:

The house's smallest sound prevents falling asleep and overwhelms the ability to ignore it.

Every movement is distractive, no matter how small.

Many odors, which others barely note, cause people with ADHD to leave the room.

Individuals with ADHD have continually disturbed their lives through events that are not common to the neurotypical. Such interruption enforces the ADHD person's perception of being weird, prickly, challenging, and high-maintenance. But that's all people with ADHD have ever heard about. It's common for them. The notion of being special, and that distinction viewed by others as unfair, is made a part of how they are treated. It's part of your identity.

A person with ADHD can sometimes hit the do-or-die deadline and produce lots of high-quality work in a short time. The entire semester of study is compressed into a single hyper focused night of perfection. Many people with ADHD are causing challenges to create the energy to activate them and make them work. High-intensity emergencies are managed with ease by the "masters of disasters," only to fall apart when things again become normal.

Nevertheless, going from crisis to crisis is a tough way of living life. Occasionally I come into people using frustration to get the rush of adrenaline they need to participate and be successful. We revive resentments or slights, to inspire themselves from years ago. The price they pay is so high for their productivity that they can be seen as having personality disorders.

Why aren't people with ADHD getting things done?

People with ADHD are both mystified and frustrated by the ADHD brain's secrets, namely the intermittent ability to be super-focused when interested and challenged and unable to initiate and sustain personal boring projects. It's not that they don't want to do anything, or that they can't do the job. We know that they are strong and smart because many times, they have proven it. The lifelong frustration is never to be sure that when needed when anticipated when others count on them, they will be able to engage. When people with ADHD see themselves as undependable, they begin to doubt their talents and feel the shame of being unreliable.

Mood and level of energy often swing with varying interests and challenges. The person with ADHD is lethargic, quarrelsome, and filled with frustration when bored, unengaged, or stuck by a job.

Why our ADHD motors always run?

By the time adolescents are most individuals with ADHD, their physical hyperactivity has been pushed inside and hidden. But it's there, and it still impairs the potential of participating at the moment, listening to other people, relaxing enough to fall asleep at night, and getting peace periods.

Therefore, as stimulant treatment brings distractibility and impulsivity back to normal levels, an individual with ADHD may not be able to use his or her healed state. He's always powered forward as if shielded from the rest of the world by a motor on the inside. Through puberty, most people with nervous systems in the ADHD type have developed the necessary social skills to cover up the lack of them.

Yet they rarely completely get away with it. The world has moved on without them as they turn back into what has happened while they were lost in their thoughts. Uh-oh. They're lost and don't know what's happening, what they've missed, and what's expected of them now. It is uncomfortable and disorienting to re-enter the neurotypical environment. The outside world is not as vivid to people with ADHD as the fantastic ideas they've had while trapped in their own thoughts.

Why organization confuses people with ADHD?

The Mind of ADHD is a large, unorganized library. This includes masses of knowledge but not whole books in fragments. The information exists in many forms— such as posts, images, audio clips, web pages — and also in ways and opinions that nobody ever had before. Nevertheless, there is no catalog of cards, and the "books" are not arranged by issue or even alphabetized.

Each person with ADHD has their own brain library and their own way of storing an enormous amount of material. No wonder the average person with ADHD is unable at the moment to find the correct piece of information— there is no effective method for finding it. Important items (God help us, significant to somebody else) have no fixed place, and could also be invisible or entirely missing. For example, the child with ADHD comes home and tells Mom he doesn't have to do homework. He watches television or plays video games until his bedtime. Later, in the morning, he remembers having a major report due. Was the child lying to the parent, knowingly, or was he really unaware of the important task?

For a person with ADHD, the out-of-sight knowledge and memories are out of view. Her mind is a machine in RAM, with no secure access to information on the hard drive.

Working memory is the capacity to have data in one's head and to be able to manipulate the data in order to come up with a response or action plan. A person's mind with ADHD is full of life's minutiae ("Where are my keys?" "Where have I parked the car?"), so little space for fresh thoughts and memories is left over. In order to make room for new information something has to be discarded or forgotten. Many people with ADHD need for knowledge are in their brain... somewhere. It's simply not available on request.

Why don't we see clearly?

People have little self-awareness in the world of ADHD. While they are often able to read other people well, it is difficult for the average person with ADHD to realize from moment to moment how they are doing themselves, the impact they are having on others, and how they feel about it. Neurotypicals view that as callous, selfish, unscrupulous, or socially inept. Taken together, a person with ADHD's susceptibility to other people's negative opinions, and the lack of momentary ability to observe oneself, create a witch's brew.

If a person can't see what's happening right now, the feedback loop he's learning from is broken. If a person doesn't know what's wrong or how bad it's wrong, then he doesn't know how to fix it. When people with ADHD do not know what they do well, they will not do more. They're not learning from the practice.

The ADHD mind's inability to discern how things go has many implications:

> Several individuals with ADHD think the input they get from others is different from what they interpret. Several times (and often too late), they find out that the other people were right all along. It is not until something goes wrong that

they can see and grasp what was clear to everyone else. Instead, they come to believe they cannot trust their own understanding of what is happening. They lose confidence in themselves. Even though they argue that there are many people with ADHD who are never sure they are right about anything.

> The effects of treatment may not be understood by people with ADHD, even when those benefits are apparent. If a patient sees neither the ADHD problems nor the treatment benefits, he finds no reason to continue treatment.

> People with ADHD sometimes see themselves as being underestimated, unappreciated, and targeted for no cause whatsoever. Alienation is a hot topic. Some assume that only someone else with ADHD will actually "see" them.

Why individuals with ADHD are time challenged?

Since people with ADHD have no accurate sense of time, it is all happening right now or not at all. There also has to be the idea of time along with the concept of ordination (what must be performed first; what must come second). The item at the top of the list has to be finished first, and the whole job has to be completed with time left.

I noticed that 85 percent of my ADHD patients are not wearing a watch or owning it. It was not used by more than half of those who wore a watch, but wore it as a necklace, or not to hurt the feelings of the person who gave it. To people with ADHD, time is an irrational concept. Some things seem important, but people with ADHD never got the hang of it.

1.4: ADHD in women

Females mostly live with undiagnosed attention-deficit / hyperactivity disorder (ADHD), mostly because it's a condition that has traditionally been thought to affect mostly males, but also because females tend to have a less obvious type than males. At school, girls ' ADHD symptoms may be overlooked because females are more likely to have inattentive ADHD, which usually does not have visible behavioral problems that hyperactive/impulsive ADHD does.

A girl with ADHD may be known as Chatty Cathy— the friendly school-age girl who tells friends stories all the time. Or she might be the daydreamer— the intelligent, nervous girl with the disorganized locker.

But what happens with growing up? And when she is not diagnosed with ADHD until she is a woman? Was her perspective different from what ADHD people are experiencing?

ADHD has not been researched extensively in women. Much more is learned about how children are affected. But some patterns seem to differ with ADHD between men and women.

Women, Men, and ADHD

Individual problems with ADHD have to parallel those in the entire population, says Stephanie Sarkis, Ph.D., a psychotherapist in Boca Raton, Fla.

For example, she says men with ADHD tend to experience more car accidents, school suspensions, substance abuse, and rage and behavioral issues than women with ADHD. But men, regardless of ADHD, are generally more prone to these kinds of issues.

ADHD women are more likely to eating disorders, obesity, low self-esteem, depression, and anxiety. But they do so in the general population.

Such problems often also play out in various aspects of their lives. Anthony Rostain, MD, professor of psychiatry and paediatrics at the University of Pennsylvania School of Medicine, says men with ADHD may have problems at work, unable to complete their tasks, or get angry too quickly at subordinates.

In contrast, women are more likely to see conflicts at home. Kathleen Nadeau, Ph.D., clinical psychologist, and director of Maryland's Chesapeake ADHD Center in Silver Spring, says her female ADHD patients, particularly mothers, come to her in a "constant overwhelming condition." "Society has some set of expectations that we put on women, and ADHD sometimes makes them more difficult to meet," Nadeau says. She points to the traditional roles of women in society. "They are meant to be the household manager, planner, and primary parent. It is expected that women will recall birthdays and anniversaries, and do laundry and keep track of events. That's all hard for an ADHD individual.'

Roots in Childhood

Many women with ADHD have long recounted having these problems. "A lot of women tell me they'd look straight at the teacher (in school), so they didn't get into trouble but didn't know what was going on," Nadeau says. "They do not work well, but they are strong... Their signs are more subtle. "ADHD is one of the most commonly diagnosed behavioral disorders in children and is a chronic condition that often persists for life. It affects an estimated 3 to 9 percent of U.S. youth.

Hyperactivity, lack of focus, and impulsive behavior are the hallmarks of ADHD.

But different shades of ADHD do exist. The most noticeable is the hyperactive-impulsive type, in which children have trouble sitting still and completing tasks like work at school. We may be overly emotional or spill inappropriate comments out at random. Another form of ADHD is inattentive, with symptoms such as lack of focus, forgetfulness, fatigue, organizational difficulty, and daydreaming.

Although there are always some exceptions to the rule, many experts say that boys tend more towards hyperactive-impulsive symptoms, and girls are more inclined towards inattentive symptoms. "Females tend to be more of an inattentive type and unconsciously overwhelmed by emotions, and guys tend to be more hyperactive," says Fran Walfish, doctor, child, and adult psychotherapist in Beverly Hills, Calif. "I've seen dreamy boys and hyperactive girls, but these are the exceptions."

Later Diagnosis

Often, women's ADHD gets overlooked before college, when they start showing a lack of self-regulation and self-management, Rostain says.

"Risks to them include issues like being affected by a sorority or the drug scene for fun," he says. "And they're not as crazy as the guys [with ADHD] but more risk-taking compared to other girls." ADHD's underlying mechanisms are the same for males and females. Both have difficulty in planning, coordinating, recalling the specifics, and paying attention.

But where the gender differences often lie, is how ADHD plays out in symptoms. And the explanation for that is possibly a social one.

Because inattention is much more subtle than hyperactivity, this may be the reason why boys are almost three times more likely to be diagnosed with ADHD than girls. However, by the time that gap reaches adulthood, it shrinks to two by one. This is possible because girls, relative to boys, are often diagnosed later in life.

Girls may "slip through the cracks" and be diagnosed later, says Walfish, because their ADHD symptoms might be covered up.

Women with ADHD: When Life Overwhelms

Responsibilities like family and work can make it hard for women to cover up or handle ADHD. But there are certain things women can do to cope with the demands of life.

Nadeau suggests ensuring that family and friends understand ADHD so that they are more accepting and have realistic expectations. Women should also simplify whenever possible: reduce unnecessary pressures and responsibilities and discuss activities that most challenge them with their family and partner.

It can also help hire a professional organizer or work with a coach to develop good habits and systems of organization. One of the items Sarkis suggests is hiring an assistant who can come in to do light cleaning for 6 to 8 hours a week, go through documents, and help organize things.

"I've got people telling me it's going to be too expensive, and it may be, but people with ADHD can't afford no help," says Sarkis.

1.5: Symptoms of ADHD in women

Women's ADHD symptoms are often described as ADHD symptoms in girls are often explained as character traits instead of ADHD. For instance, you might think of a girl as spacey, a daydreamer, forgetful, or chatty. A woman may reach out for help with her ADHD later in life, only to be diagnosed with depression or anxiety instead. The good thing is that people are getting more aware of ADHD symptoms, which means women are able to get the help they need.

Women with ADHD face the same frustrated and tired feelings that men with ADHD might feel. Psychological distress, insufficient emotions, low self-esteem, and chronic stress are all normal. Many women with ADHD believe their lives are out of control or in turmoil, and daily tasks may seem incredibly enormous.

Although many women are expected to be caregivers, for a woman with ADHD, this task can be extremely difficult. If things feel out of control, and she has trouble managing and preparing her own life, it seems almost impossible to take care of others. This position may also greatly enhance her feelings of inadequacy.

Common Signs of ADHD in Women

Here are some ways that ADHD might show up in your life:

• The work desk is stacked high with paperwork. Even if you're making a big effort to clean things up, it just remains clear for a day or two.

• It feels difficult to be in the workplace. The noise and the people make it difficult to get the work done.

• Sometimes you stay in the office late, because the only time you can work well is when everyone else has left, and it's quiet.

• You spend a great deal of time and effort looking "natural," and hope that no one will recognize the real you.

• You feel like being lost in the paper. In your car, at work, at home, and even in your purse. You have an uncomfortable feeling that unpaid bills and unfinished tasks disappear under the paper.

• You don't like to go to parties or other social gatherings, because they make you feel nervous and shy.

• Unless you're the one talking or it's a subject you find really interesting, the mind drifts during the conversations.

• Friendships can be hard to navigate, as social rules seem confusing.

• You speak more than anybody you meet.

• You've always been described as a tomboy growing up because you had so much energy, and you liked to be busy.

• You don't feel prepared with money, and usually, bills are behind you.

• Often you overspend to offset other problems. You don't have, for example, a clean outfit to wear for an office party, so you buy a new one. Or you've missed someone's birthday, so you're buying an expensive gift to make up for it.

- Shopping trips make you feel better at the moment, but later on, you feel sorry when the credit card bill comes in.

- You spend a lot of time, money, and product research to help you organize yourself better, but then you don't use them.

- You feel very reluctant to have people visit your home because it's so disorganized and cluttered.

- You wish that you could be a better friend, wife, or mom, and you'd do the things other people are doing. You wish you could recall birthdays, bake cookies, for example, and arrive on time for a wedding.

- If you can't do the things society expects women to do, people might think you don't care.

- You are confused by the grocery stores, and you find it difficult to make choices about what to purchase.

- A key ingredient for a meal is often forgotten even if you take longer in the supermarket than most people.

- It seems as if every day is spent responding to requests and minimizing accidents rather than pushing the goals forward.

- You feel frustrated that even though you know you're just as smart, people you went to school passed you by with their accomplishments.

- You are feeling overwhelming disappointment and anger that your ability has not been achieved.

- Little things can drive you over the top and make you feel emotional.

- You have difficulty in relaxing.

Many women are relieved to learn that behaviors they have so long struggled with are due to ADHD.

1.6: ADHD Statistics: ADHD in Women

About 45 percent of women diagnosed with ADHD also meet the criteria for another disorder.25 People with ADHD have a greater risk of major depression— by 2.5 times— compared to women without ADHD. Approximately 28 percent of women classified as obese also have an ADHD diagnosis.27 Women with ADHD who have not been diagnosed until adulthood are more likely to have a history of depression and anxiety than those with ADHD. Teenage girls with ADHD are more likely to: deal with emotional, attentional, and behavioral difficulties, have weaker self-conceptions, experience more psychological distress and impairment, and feel less in control of their lives.

Chapter 2: Impact and treatment

Knowledge of ADHD in adult women at this time is extremely limited, as little research on this demographic has been performed. Females have only recently started to be diagnosed and treated for ADHD, and today, most of what we learn about this demographic is focused on the clinical experience of mental health professionals who specialize in treating women.

2.1: Impact of ADHD in women

ADHD is often overlooked in young girls, the reasons remaining unclear, and many females are not diagnosed until they are adults. Often a woman comes to recognize her own ADHD after a diagnosis has been made to one of her children. As she learns more about ADHD, she starts seeing in herself many similar patterns.

Some women are seeking treatment for ADHD because their lives are out of control— their finances may be in chaos; their paperwork and record-keeping are mostly poorly managed; they may struggle unsuccessfully to fulfill the demands of their jobs; and they may feel even less able to keep up with the daily tasks of food, laundry, and life management. Other women are more effective at suppressing their ADHD, struggling valiantly to keep up with increasingly difficult demands by working in the night, and wasting their free time trying to "get organized." But whether a woman's life is obviously in turmoil, or whether she can conceal her problems, she always describes herself as feeling overwhelmed and tired.

While ADHD research in women continues to lag behind that in adult males, many clinicians find significant concerns in women with ADHD and co-existing conditions. In women with ADHD, there may be compulsive overeating, alcohol abuse, and chronic sleep deprivation.

Women with ADHD often experience dysphoria (unpleasant mood), major depression, and anxiety disorders, with rates of depressive disorders and anxiety similar to those of men with ADHD. Women with ADHD, however, appear to have more psychological distress and a lower self-image than men with ADHD.

In contrast with women without ADHD, women who are diagnosed with ADHD in adulthood are more likely to have depressive symptoms, are more stressed and anxious, have more external control locations (tendency to assign performance and problems to external factors such as chance), have less self-esteem and are more interested in emotion-oriented coping strategies (use self-protective measures to reduce s).

Studies show that ADHD causes stress to the whole family within a family member. For women, however, stress levels may be higher than for men, because they assume more responsibility for the home and children. However, recent research suggests that women's husbands with ADHD are less forgiving of ADHD traits in their partner than men's wives with ADHD. Chronic stress takes its toll on people with ADHD and physically and psychologically affects them. Women who suffer from chronic stress, such as that associated with ADHD are more at risk for chronic stress-related diseases such as fibromyalgia.

Thus, it becomes increasingly clear that a significant public health concern is the lack of adequate identification and treatment of ADHD in women.

2.2: The challenge of receiving appropriate treatment

ADHD is a disorder that affects many aspects of mood, cognitive abilities, behaviors, and everyday life. A multimodal approach that involves medication, psychotherapy, stress management, as well as ADHD coaching and/or professional organization that includes effective treatment for ADHD in adult women.

Even those women who are fortunate enough to receive a specific diagnosis of ADHD still face the corresponding challenge of finding a doctor who can provide the proper treatment. There are very few physicians who are experienced in the management of adult ADHD and even fewer who are familiar with the unique problems that women with ADHD face. As a result, most clinicians use standard approaches to psychotherapy. While these methods can be helpful in providing insight into emotional and behavioral problems, they don't help a woman with ADHD learn how to manage her ADHD on a daily basis better or learn strategies to live a more successful and satisfying life.

ADHD-focused therapies have been developed to address a wide range of issues, including self-esteem, interpersonal and family issues, daily health habits, day-to-day stress, and life-management abilities. Such interventions are referred to as "neurocognitive psychotherapy," combining cognitive behavioral therapy with techniques for cognitive rehabilitation. Cognitive-behavioral therapy focuses on the psychological issues of ADHD (e.g., self-esteem, self-acceptance, self-blame), while the cognitive recovery approach focuses on life management skills to develop cognitive functions (remembering, thinking, comprehension, and problem-solving, analyzing, and using judgment), learning compensatory methods, and environmental adjustment.

2.3: Medication management in women with ADHD

Medication problems are often more complicated for women with ADHD compared with men. Any approach to medicine needs to take into account all facets of the woman's life, including treating co-existing conditions. Women with ADHD are more likely to suffer from co-existing anxiety and/or depression and from a range of other conditions, including learning disabilities. Because alcohol and drug use disorders are common in women with ADHD and can occur at an early age, a careful history of substance use is essential.

Hormone fluctuations throughout the menstrual cycle and throughout the lifespan (e.g., puberty, perimenopause, and menopause) may further complicate medication with an increase in ADHD symptoms whenever estrogen levels fall. Hormone replacement may, in some cases, need to be added into the medication regimen used to treat ADHD.

For more information on managing medication in adults with ADHD, see Managing Medication.

2.4: Other treatment approaches

Women with ADHD could benefit from one or more of the following approaches to treatment:

1. Training with parents. In most families, the mother is the primary parent. It is expected that mothers will be the household and family manager— roles requiring attention, coordination, and preparation, as well as the ability to play multiple responsibilities. Nonetheless, ADHD usually interferes with those abilities, making mother's job much more difficult for women with ADHD.

For a fact, since ADHD is inherited, a woman with ADHD is more likely to have a child with ADHD than a woman without the condition, thus further raising her parental difficulties. Women may need parental and household management training that is geared to adults with ADHD. Often recommended for parents with ADHD are evidence-based parent intervention interventions that are shown to be beneficial in children with ADHD.

However, research on these parent training approaches has indicated that if the mother has high levels of ADHD symptoms, parent training may be less effective. Therefore, the integration of life management strategies for adult ADHD into parent training programs for mothers with ADHD may be appropriate.

2. Group treatment. Social issues develop early for women with ADHD and appear to increase with age. People with ADHD have greater problems with self-esteem than men with ADHD, and often feel shame as compared to women without ADHD.

Because many women with ADHD feel shame and rejection, psychotherapy groups specifically designed for women with ADHD can provide a therapeutic experience— a place where other women can feel understood and accepted, and a safe place to start their journey towards accepting themselves more and learning how to manage their lives better.

3. Coaching ADHD. ADHD coaching, a new profession, has evolved in response to the need for structure, support, and focus among some adults with ADHD. Coaching is often done over the phone or by e-mail

4. Organizing professionals. When contemporary life has become increasingly complicated, the profession of organizers has evolved to meet the demand. People with ADHD usually struggle in many areas of their lives against very high levels of disorganization. Many women may keep order at work but at the expense of an orderly household. Disorganization is common for others and increases ADHD's challenges and difficulties.

A qualified organizer can provide hands-on assistance in organizing, discarding, filing, and storing items in a home or office to help set up more easily maintainable structures.

5. Guidance on the career. Just as women with ADHD may need specific guidance as a parent with ADHD, they may also benefit greatly from career guidance that can help them harness their strengths and minimize the impact of ADHD on workplace performance. Most technical and office jobs involve the very activities and duties that are most difficult for an ADHD person, including paying attention to detail, scheduling, paperwork, and maintaining an orderly workspace.

Sometimes a career or job change is needed to reduce the intense daily stress that most individuals with ADHD often experience in the workplace. A career specialist who has experience with ADHD can provide useful advice.

2.5: Ways that women with ADHD can help themselves

Working first with a therapist to develop better life and stress management techniques is beneficial for a female with ADHD. However, without the guidance of a therapist, coach, or organizer, the following strategies can be used at home to reduce the impact of ADHD:

• Instead of judging and blaming yourself, understand and accept your ADHD challenges;

• Recognized the sources of stress in your daily life, and make life changes systematically to reduce your stress level.

• Make life simpler.

• Have family and friends look for structure and support.

Get advice from parenting experts.

• Build a family that is ADHD friendly, and that cooperates and respects one another.

• Plan your own routine timeouts.

• Develop healthy self-care routines such as adequate sleep and exercise, and good nutrition.

• Focus on the stuff you love.

Individuals with ADHD, depending on their gender, age, and environment, have different needs and challenges. Unrecognized and untreated, the effects of ADHD may be important for mental health and education. It is very important for women with ADHD to receive an accurate diagnosis that addresses both the symptoms and other important functioning and impairment issues, helping to determine appropriate treatment and strategies for the individual woman with ADHD.

Chapter 3: Neurodiversity

Neurodiversity is the idea that differences in neurology are the result of normal, natural variations in the human genome. They don't need a cure. Instead, they need assistance and accommodation. Organizations, where such accommodations are made by leaders, reap tremendous benefits. Common disorders falling within this category include autistic spectrum disorders, dyspraxia, dyslexia, and, among others, attention deficit hyperactivity disorder (ADHD).

To me, the idea of neurodiversity is that neurological differences such as autism and ADHD result from normal, natural variation of the human genome. It represents a new and fundamentally different way of looking at conditions that have historically been pathologized; it is a point of view that is not universally accepted even though research is gradually supporting it.

That science suggests conditions such as autism have stable prevalence as far back as we can measure in human society. They understand that autism, ADHD, and other disorders occur through a combination of genetic predisposition and contact with the environment; they are not the result of illness or injury.

At the same time, we identify diseases and injuries (physical and environmental) that will result in brain injuries that look very similar to autism and other differences in their effects. Acceptance of neurodiversity certainly does not only include passive acceptance of such injury and insult, although we should accept individuals so impacted unconditionally.

Smallpox is a disease that attacks healthy people; by understanding its foundations, and planning an attack at that level, one can seek its eradication. At that basic level, autism — as a permanent part of a normally healthy person — can be recognized. But if it is an innate part of the individual, it is not subject to the same simplistic manner of attacking and cure.

That's why it is such an incredibly complex challenge to remediate its medical complications.

Indeed, many people who embrace the concept of neurodiversity believe that people with differences need no cure; instead, they need help and accommodation.

We look at the pool of diverse society and see the range of different ideas in the center that has made the advancement of humanity possible in science and creative arts. At the margins, they see people who are mentally disabled by being "too different." When a problem is not solved by 99 neurologically similar men, it is often the one percent fellow that holds the key. Yet, most or all of the time, that person may be disabled or disadvantaged. People are disabled to supporters of neurodiversity because they're at the margins of the bell curve, not because they're ill or broken.

As a person with autism, I find the idea of natural variation more compelling than the alternative— the possibility that I'm innately bad, or defective, and requiring repair. I did not learn about my own autism until I reached middle age. All those years (pre-diagnosis), I assumed my struggles stemmed from inherent shortcomings. To claim that I am different— not flawed — is a much healthier position to take. It's even easier to know the theory is supported by science.

To many supporters of neurodiversity, "cure" talk sounds like an assault on their very being. They detest those words are for the same reason that other groups detest talking about "curing gayness" or "passing for white," and they perceive the accommodation of neurological differences as an issue of similarly charged civil rights. If their diversity is part of their make-up, they believe that it is their right to be "as-is" accepted and supported. They should not be turned into something else— especially against their will— to fit some imagined ideal for society.

The difference— and this is a big sticking point for critics of neurodiversity— is that differences in racial or sexual orientation don't physically impair an individual while differences in neurology can. The fact complicates this situation far more.

It is also worth noting that, in general, the neurodiverse looks just like anyone else.

Therefore, when we behave in an uncommon or unexpected manner, we can elicit unwanted negative reactions from an unsuspecting public. For that reason, learning the basics of getting along in a neurotypical community is important to us, all who are special. Some people see this as an unacceptable compromise, but I see it as recognizing a reality that is unchanging (or very slow to change).

There's no doubt that the neurodiversity gave a lot of great things to human society. If neurology truly enabled those successes, it follows logically that an effort to "heal" potential illness by removing our differences would be profoundly detrimental to humanity.

There is also no doubt that communities are filled with people whose talents remain hidden and whose differences keep them from living alone. Some of those individuals have differences that make them behave or act aggressively towards others. The roots of their issues remain poorly understood, but we cannot deny their existence alongside those who are endowed with a different version of what might be called "the same difference." They are deserving of significant help. I don't believe that's inconsistent with the neurodiversity ideals.

Opponents of neurodiversity look at those who are disabled by difference, and say that attributing that to "normal variation" is wrong. Unfortunately, as the evidence for neurodiversity accumulates, it seems more and more likely that an overall neurological difference cure is not possible, and if the diversity is at the root of the achievements of some people, it is not desirable either.

So, what to do in a progressive society? How can we help?

I hope we should lighten the burden of physical illness without changing the person's nature. Early speech and behavioral therapy is a prime example of this today. Society can adapt in some situations to make houses, parks, and places of work more welcoming. At the same time, we will build treatments that will help us lead our best lives possible. Furthermore, we should change attitudes towards people who are different in order to be accepted, appreciated, and made to feel part of the human community.

When we agree that a world of neurodiversity is a good world, we will have made great strides in our thinking. If only this was so fast!

Neurological disability is very true, but you feel about neurodiversity as a concept. There is not any doubt in my mind that society has a duty to relieve the suffering caused by a disability and to help people with disabilities live their best lives. I like to think that most people approve of that general idea. The real question is how to get there faster.

We made very little progress in developing therapies or treatments to remedy the worst effects of the neurological difference. We still don't know much about how different neurology impacts the rest of our body systems or our overall quality of life as we age. That — for me — is a great tragedy for our generation. In thinking about disorders such as autism as "diseases that need to be treated," we have followed a course of study that has contributed to a greater understanding of certain specifics but a very little that actually helps the broader autistic community.

I believe it is time to change direction. Rather than focusing most of our budget on fundamental genetic and biological research, let's move the focus to practical research to help today's people living with neurological disparity. Those people have a tremendous range of concerns and issues to address, so the scope of the work needed is wide.

At the same time, let's put more effort into environmental research — studies that will help us understand how we can poison people and create damage that mimics natural variation (but worsens it).

If neurological differences do indeed occur naturally, there will be no terribly productive research into foundation level cures for those differences. Having said that, in recognizing genetic variations that lead to major impairment with no clear reciprocal gain, we should consider some real breakthroughs.

Identifying such mutations and discovering causes is a significant scientific achievement. We haven't converted this research into effective treatments yet, but I see the potential. I certainly believe that such work will continue, but I also believe that our goals need to change.

Previous campaigns to recognize the diversity of race or gender were easier compared to the neurological inclusion battle that was to come. All we had to alter in them were attitudes and behaviors. For neurodiversity, we have to change assumptions while at the same time finding ways to solve critical working issues.

After many years of struggle, discriminating against someone by reason of race or faith anywhere in America is against the law. Sadly, in other places, we haven't come that far. It is still legal, in many states, to fire someone for being gay. People who act differently by virtue of their neurology have no other protections than those provided for in the Americans With Disabilities Act.

The task of changing societal attitudes is complicated by the invisibility of neurological differences. It's difficult for the general public to tolerate an unknown phenomenon that causes unpredictable actions with no obvious explanation beyond "acting badly." Many people think the recognition of neurodiversity means accepting what otherwise are socially unacceptable behaviors in the name of embracing difference. I totally do not agree with that idea. We all have to act right (ethically, morally, humanly) toward each other.

I assume that a great deal of opposition to neurodiversity stems from the (misguided) notion that embracing neurodiversity implies opposition to basic scientific research or opposition to developing tools to improve the lives of people with disabilities. I don't think it's meant or implied, either.

While still working hard to mitigate or remove its negative effects, we should accept that neurological disparity is a natural part of us. At the same time, we should recognize and accept the very real benefits that difference offers many of us and welcome people as they are because that is reality. As with any debilitating disparity, a parent may wish things were otherwise, but they are not, and the healthiest way forward is unconditional acceptance of our loved ones.

I believe that accepting neurodiversity backed by solid research on how we can be our best (the least disabled, the most productive, etc.) is the most positive position that those of us who are different can adopt. I celebrate all the people who are fighting for the rights of different people, and I look forward to the further fruits of those efforts. In the meantime, as I always have, I will use my own differences— to make a living by my neurology doing those odd things that I do better.

John Elder Robison is an autism spectrum adult and an autism parent of an adult son. He is currently a Scholar in Residence at William & Mary College in Williamsburg, VA. He is a member of the US Department of Health and Human Services ' Interagency Autism Coordinating Committee and serves on many other boards related to neuroscience. The words spoken here are his own. He's the author of 3 books — Raising Cubby, Be Different, Look Me in The Eye, and many blogs.

Where Neurodiversity Began?

In the late 1990s, Judy Singer developed the term neurodiversity. Singer, an autism spectrum sociologist, dismissed the idea that people with autism were disabled.

Singer believed that their minds function only differs from those of others. Activists in the autism community, and beyond, quickly adopted the term. It has been used by advocates to combat stigma and promote inclusion in schools and workplaces.

The movement stresses that the aim should not be to "heal" people whose brain works differently. The objective is to embrace these as part of the mainstream. And that means providing needed support so they can fully participate as members of the community.

3.1: Neurodivergent

Neurodivergent individuals–who have neurological differences, such as autism dyslexia, developmental coordination disorder, or ADHD, but not limited to. ... People whose minds and brains function in a manner considered "normal," aka neurotypical people, are privileged in relation to people who are neurodivergent.

3.2: Neurodiversity and Learning and Thinking Differences

The idea that people are learners, of course, diverse is important for children with differences in learning and thought. It can reduce the stigma and feeling that they have something "wrong." And that could help build trust, self-esteem, motivation, and resilience.

It also supports approaches to teaching, which can benefit children with differences in learning and thinking. UDL, for example, shares many of the neurodiversity concepts.

UDL acknowledges that there is a wide range of students with a wide array of skills. To remove barriers to learning, it uses a variety of teaching strategies. The aim is to give all students equal opportunities to succeed, of all abilities.

3.3: Embracing neurodiversity

In the basement of the headquarters of the Bureau International des Poids et Mesures (BIPM) in Sevres, France, a suburb of Paris, lies a piece of metal that has been secured under three bell jars in an environmentally controlled chamber since 1889. It represents the world standards for the kilogram, and all other kilo measurements all around the world must be compared with this one prototype and calibrated with it. Such a norm does not exist for the human brain.

Research as you might, there is no brain picked in a jar in the Smithsonian Museum's basement or the National Institute of Health or anywhere else in the world that represents the standard to which all other human brains must be compared. Since this is the case, how do we decide whether any human brain or mind is abnormal or normal?

Psychiatrists have their diagnostic handbooks, to be sure. But when it comes to mental disorders like autism, dyslexia, attention deficit hyperactivity disorder, intellectual disabilities, and even emotional and behavioral disorders, there seems to be significant confusion about when a human behavior dependent on neurology reaches the crucial threshold from normal human variability to disease.

A quite major cause of this ambiguity is the emergence of studies over the past two decades, which suggest that many brain or mind disorders bring both strengths and weaknesses with them. For example, people diagnosed with autism spectrum disorder (ASD) tend to have abilities related to interacting with systems (e.g., programming languages, mathematical structures, machines), and tests to find tiny details in complex patterns are stronger than control subjects.

On the nonverbal Raven's Matrices intelligence test, they also score significantly higher than on the verbal Wechsler Scales.

A practical result of this recent understanding of ASD-related abilities is that technology companies have been actively recruiting people with ASD for jobs that include systemizing activities such as computer manual writing, database management, and computer code checking for bugs.

For people with other mental disorders, important traits have also been found. Individuals with dyslexia have been shown to possess global visual-spatial capacities, including the ability to identify "impossible objects" (of the kind popularized by M. C. Escher), interpret low-definition, or blurry visual images, and more easily and effectively perceive peripheral or diffused visual information than people without dyslexia.

These visual-spatial abilities in jobs requiring three-dimensional thought such as astrophysics, molecular biology, genetics, electronics, and computer graphics may be beneficial.

Researchers have reported improved musical abilities in people with Williams syndrome, the warmth, and friendliness of individuals with Down syndrome, and the caring activities of people with Prader-Willi syndrome, in the area of intellectual disabilities.

Researchers have finally observed that subjects with attention deficit hyperactivity disorder (ADHD) and bipolar disorder display higher levels of novelty-seeking and creativity than matched controls.

Such strengths might suggest an evolutionary explanation for why the gene pool still contains these disorders. An increasing number of scientists suggest that psychopathologies in the past, as well as in the present, could have conferred specific evolutionary advantages.

The systemizing capabilities of individuals with autism spectrum disorder could have been highly adaptive to prehistoric human survival. As autism activist Temple Grandin, who has autism herself, surmised: "The first stone spear was developed by some guy with high-functioning Asperger's; it was not developed by the social ones yakking around the campfire."

Similarly, in preliterate cultures, the three-dimensional thinking seen in some people with dyslexia may have been highly adaptive in designing tools, plotting hunting routes and building shelters, and would not have been considered a barrier to learning.

The main signs of ADHD, including hyperactivity, distractibility, and impulsivity, would have been adaptive traits in hunting and gathering societies where people who were peripatetic in their search for food, fast in their response to environmental stimuli, and deft in moving towards or away from potential prey would have thrived.

There could also have been evolutionary advantages for people with mania in prehistoric times, as high energy and creative expression could have enhanced sexual and reproductive success.

The cumulative effect of these studies suggests that a more judicious approach to the treatment of mental disorders would be to replace a paradigm of "disability" or "illness" with a perspective of "diversity" taking into account both strengths and weaknesses, and the idea that variation can be positive in itself. To that end, within the autism advocacy culture, a new term has emerged: neurodiversity. Although the origin of the neurodiversity movement is often traced back to a speech entitled "Don't Mourn for Us," given at the 1993 International Conference on Autism in Toronto by autism activist Jim Sinclair, the word itself was first used by autism advocates Judy Singer and New York journalist Harvey Blume to articulate it the needs of people with autism who did not want to be defined by an autism.

 Since then, the use of the word has continued to grow in areas such as disability research, special education, higher education, industry, therapy, and medicine beyond the movement of autism rights.

To accept the idea of neurodiversity will bring the study of mental health disorders into line with developments surrounding biodiversity and the cultural diversity which have already taken place over the past 50 years.

As Harvey Blume observed, "Neurodiversity can be just as important to the human race as biodiversity is to live in general. Who can tell at any given moment what sort of cabling would prove best? "How ridiculous it would be to mark a calla lily as having a" petal deficiency disorder "or to diagnose a person from the Netherlands as suffering from an" altitude deprivation syndrome. Likewise, we will agree that there is no normal brain or mind.

Chapter 4: Break barriers and conquering chaos

If you have attention deficit hyperactivity disorder (ADHD), previously known as ADD, it can seem daunting anything from paying the bills on time to keeping up with work, family, and social demands. ADHD can present challenges to adults across all areas of life and can be rough on your wellbeing as well as on-the-job and personal relations. You can experience extreme procrastination, difficulty meeting deadlines, and impulsive behavior with your symptoms. Besides, you may feel friends and family don't understand what you're up against.

Luckily there are some skills you can learn to help manage your ADHD symptoms. You will strengthen your daily habits, learn to recognize and use your strengths, and build strategies that will help you work more efficiently, retain the structure, and better communicate with others. It may also be part of helping yourself to educate others to help them understand what you are going through.

Yet improvement will not happen overnight. Such approaches for self-help for ADHD include repetition, persistence, and, perhaps most importantly, a positive attitude. But by using these methods, you can become more successful, disciplined, and in control of your life–and increase your sense of self-worth.

4.1: Self-help myth and adult ADHD

Myth: The only way to resolve my ADHD is through medication.

Fact: While medication can help some people handle the ADHD symptoms, it is not a cure, nor is it the only solution. It should be used, if used at all, in conjunction with other drugs or self-help strategies.

Myth: ADHD means that I am lazy or unintelligent, so I cannot help myself.

Fact: The effects of ADHD might have caused you and others to label you this way, but the truth is, you're not unmotivated or unintelligent— you have a disorder that interferes with some normal functions. In reality, adults with ADHD often need to find very clever ways to counteract their condition.

Myth: A health care professional will fix all of my issues with ADHD.

Fact: Healthcare professionals can help you manage ADHD symptoms, but they can do just that much. You are the one who deals with the challenges, so you are the one who can make the most of it in solving them.

Myth: ADHD is a life sentence — I'll suffer from its effects all the time.

Fact: Although there is no remedy for ADHD, there's a lot you can do to the issues that it can cause. You can find that controlling your symptoms is second nature once you become used to using techniques to support yourself.

ADHD can cause problems in all aspects of your life. But these tips will help you cope with symptoms, concentrate on yourself, and keep uncertainty calm.

4.2: Ways to get organized and controlling clutters

ADHD's signature symptoms are inattention and distractiveness— making coordination maybe the biggest challenge facing adults with the condition. If you have ADHD, the idea of getting organized will leave you feeling stressed, whether it's at work or at home.

Nonetheless, you should learn to break down the activities into smaller steps and follow a structured organizational approach. You can set up yourself to maintain order and manage clutter by introducing various structures and routines and taking advantage of tools such as regular planners and reminders.

Develop good and neat habits:

Begin by categorizing your items, determining which are important and which can be stored or discarded to organize a room, home, or office. To organize yourself, get used to taking notes and composing lists. Keep your newly structured system running normal, daily routines.

Create rooms. Ask yourself on a daily basis what you need, and consider storage bins or closets for items that you don't. Designate specific areas for objects that can easily be lost, such as keys, bills, and other items. Throw things away, which you don't need.

Use a day planner or calendar app. using a day planner or a calendar on your smartphone or computer effectively will help you remember appointments and deadlines. You can also set up automatic reminders with electronic calendars, so scheduled events don't slip your mind off.

Utilize lists. To keep the track of regularly scheduled tasks, projects, deadlines, and appointments, use the lists and notes. When you decide to use a daily schedule, keep all lists and notes inside. You also have multiple use options on your smartphone or computer. Look for Applications or Project Managers "to do."

Now deal with it. Through filing papers, cleaning up messes, or answering phone calls promptly, you will prevent forgetfulness, clutter, and procrastination, not sometime in the future. If a mission can be completed in two minutes or less, instead of putting it off for later, do it on the spot.

Tame your paper trail:

If you have ADHD, the paperwork could constitute a big part of your disorganization. But the endless stacks of mail and papers were strewn around your kitchen, desk, or office can be avoided. All it takes is some time to set up a system of paperwork that works for you.

Deal on a daily basis with the post. Set aside to deal with the mail a few minutes each day, preferably as soon as you put it inside. It helps to have a dedicated spot where you can collect the mail and either dump it, file it, or act on it.

Leave empty-handed. Minimize the amount of paper you'll need to handle: electronic demand statements and no paper copies of payments. You can reduce junk mail in the USA by opting out of the Mail Preference Service of the Direct Marketing Association (DMA).

Establish a filing system. Use separate file folders or dividers for various types of documents (such as medical records, receipts, and income statements). Mark and color-code your files, so you can quickly find out what you need.

4.3: Tips for managing your time and staying on schedule

Time management problems are typical symptoms of ADHD. Sometimes you can lose track of time, miss deadlines, procrastinate, and underestimate how much time you need to perform tasks, or find yourself doing things in the wrong order. Many adult females with ADHD spend so much time on one task— called "hyper focusing "— that nothing else is done. These may leave you feeling frustrated and inept and may make others impatient. There are, however, solutions to help you manage your time better.

Time management:

Adults with a disability and attention deficit often have a different perception of how time goes by. Use the oldest trick in the book to sync your sense of time with everybody else: one clock.

Become a Watchman of the Clock. Use a wristwatch or wall or desk clock, which is highly visible to help keep track of time. Create a note of the time that you start a job by saying it out loud or by writing it down.

Use those timers. Allocate limited time for each task, and use a timer or alarm to alert you when the time is up. Consider setting the alarm to go off at regular intervals for longer tasks to keep you productive and aware of how much time passes.

Contribute more time to yourself than you think you need. Adults with ADHD are notoriously bad at predicting how long something will take. Give yourself a break by adding 10 minutes for every thirty minutes of time you think it will take you to get someplace or complete a mission.

Plan early and create reminders. Write down the levels fifteen minutes earlier than they really are. Set up reminders to make sure you leave on time and make sure you've got everything you need in advance so that when it's time to go, you don't frenziedly scramble for your keys or phone.

Prioritizing tips:

Due to the fact that adults with ADHD often struggle with impulse control and jump from one subject to another, tasks can be difficult to complete, and large projects may seem overwhelming. To overcome this:

Decide first what to tackle. Tell yourself what is the most important task to do, then order the other goals after that.

Take one thing at a time. Break big projects or jobs down into smaller, manageable steps.

Stick to the plan. Avoid side tracking by sticking to your plan, using a timer to enforce it when needed.

Learn to say No:

Impulsivity can cause adults with ADHD to commit to too many work-related projects or participate in too many social engagements. But a jam-packed schedule will leave you feeling stressed, overwhelmed, and affect your work quality. Saying no to other obligations will improve your ability to perform activities, maintain social dates, and lead a healthier lifestyle. Always test the timeline before you commit to something different.

4.4: Ideas for managing bills and accounts

Managing money requires budgeting, planning, and organization, so this can pose a real challenge for many adults with ADHD. Many common money management systems don't tend to work with ADHD for adults because they require too much time, paper, and attention to detail. But if you create your own system that is both straightforward and consistent, you can get on top of your finances and put an end to over-spending, overdue bills, and penalties for missed deadlines.

Control budget:

The very first step to getting budgeting under control is an honest assessment of your financial situation. Start by keeping track of every cost for a month, no matter how small. That will enable you to analyze effectively where your money is going. You may be shocked at how much you spend on unnecessary items and purchases with an impulse. A snapshot of your spending habits can then be used to build a monthly budget based on your income and needs.

Find a way of avoiding straying from your target. For example, if you spend too much on restaurants, you can make a meal plan and a time factor for shopping and preparing meals.

Set up easy money management and bill system:

Establish a simple, structured system that helps you save papers, collect receipts, and stay on top of bills. For a person with ADHD, the chance to handle computer banking can be the gift that continues to give. This means fewer papers, no messy handwriting, and no lost slips.

Switch to banking online. Signing up for online banking can turn a thing of the past into the hit-or-miss process of balancing your budget. Your online account will list all deposits and payments, automatically tracking your balance to the penny, every day. You can also set up automatic payments for your regular monthly bills, and sign in to pay periodic and occasional bills as needed — the best part: no lost or late envelopes.

Set up reminders on bill pay. When you choose not to set up automatic payments, email reminders can still make the bill paying process simpler. You can set up text or email reminders via online banking, or schedule them in your calendar app.

Use the technology to their benefit. Free services will help you keep track of your accounts and your finances. They typically take some time to set up, but they will automatically update once you've connected your accounts. These instruments will simplify your financial life.

Stop impulse shopping:

ADHD and Shopping Impulsivity can be a quite dangerous combination. It can put you in debt, and make you feel ashamed and guilty. With a few proactive strategies, you can avoid impulsive buyouts.

· Just cash shop-leave your check book and credit cards at home.

· Cut out any credit card except one. Make a list of what you need while shopping, and stick to it.

· When shopping, use a calculator to keep a running total (hint: there is one on your mobile phone).

· Keep away from the places where you are likely to spend too much money, throw away catalogues when they come in, and block retailer emails.

4.5: Tips for staying focused and productive at work

ADHD is capable of creating special challenges at work. The tasks you may consider toughest — organization, job completion, sitting still, listening quietly — are the very things you're frequently asked to do throughout the day.

Juggling ADHD and a challenging job is not an easy task, but you can take advantage of your strengths by tailoring your workplace environment while minimizing the negative impact of your ADHD symptoms.

Get organized:

Organize your office, dressing room, or desk, one simple step at a time. Use the following methods to remain smooth and organized:

Set aside the organization's daily time. Set aside 5 to 10 minutes every day to clear your desk and arrange your paperwork. Experiment with storing things inside your desk or in bins so that your office is not cluttered as unwanted distractions.

Using colors and mailing lists. For people with ADHD, color coding can be very useful. Manage forgetfulness by writing down all of this.

Setting priorities. More essential tasks should be put on your to-do list first so that you know to do them before tasks of lower priority. Set deadlines for everything, even if imposed on themselves.

End distractions:

When you have issues of focus, where you are focused, and what's around, you can have a significant impact on how much you can get done. Let your colleagues know you need to focus and try to minimize distractions by using the following techniques:

Everywhere you work matters. If you don't have your own space, you might be able to take your job to a vacant office or meeting room. If you are in a conference or lecture hall, try sitting next to the speaker and away from the people chatting during the meeting.

Minimize commotion from outside. Face your desk to a wall and keep your office safe from noise. You could even hang up a "Do Not Disturb" sign to prevent interruptions. When possible, let your phone calls be picked up by voicemail and returned later, turn off email and social media during certain periods of the day or even fully log off the internet. Try noise-canceling headphones or a sound machine when noise distracts you.

Save big ideas for later on. All those brilliant ideas or random thoughts that continue to pop up in your head and confuse you? For later consideration, announce them on paper or on your mobile. Many people with ADHD like to plan the time to go through all the notes they've made at the end of the day.

Stretch your attention time:

You're able to focus as an adult with ADHD — it's just that you may have a hard time keeping that focus, especially when the activity isn't one you find particularly exciting about. Boring meetings or seminars are hard on anyone, but they can present a particular challenge for adults with ADHD. Likewise, those with ADHD may also have difficulty following multiple directions. To boost your concentration and ability to follow directions, use these tips:

Get it in writing. When you attend a meeting, lecture, workshop, or another event that requires close attention, ask for an advance copy of the related materials— such as a meeting agenda or overview of a lecture. Use the written notes at the meeting to guide you by active listening and taking notes. Reading, as you listen, will help you stay focused on the words of the speaker.

Echo instructions. Repeat them aloud after someone gives verbal instructions to make sure you've got it right.

Keep moving. So, stop restlessness and fidgeting, go ahead and move around–in the right places at the appropriate times. For example, try squeezing a stress ball during a meeting so long as you are not disturbing others. But walking or even jumping up and down during a break at a meeting might help you pay attention later.

4.6: Ways for managing stress and boosting mood.

Because of the impulsiveness and disorganization that often accompany ADHD, you may be dealing with irregular sleep, an unhealthy diet, or the consequences of too little exercise — all problems that can lead to extra stress, bad moods, and feeling out of hand. The best way to stop this process is to take responsibility for your lifestyle habits and create healthy new routines.

Eating right, having plenty of sleep, and regular exercise will help you stay calm, reduce mood swings, and fight off any anxiety and depression symptoms. Healthier habits can also reduce symptoms of ADHD, such as inattention, hyperactivity, and destructiveness, whereas daily activities can help make your life more manageable.

Spend time outdoors and exercise:

Working out is perhaps the most optimistic and beneficial means of reducing ADHD hyperactivity and inattention. Exercise can relieve stress, boost your mood, and calm your mind, helping to offset the excess energy and aggression that can interfere with relationships and stable feelings.

Take daily workout. Choose something strenuous and fun with which you can stick, like a team sport or work out with a friend.

Improve stress relief by outdoor exercise— people with ADHD also benefit from the sunlight and the green environment.

Try relaxing workout types, including mindful walking, yoga, or Tai chi. besides relieving stress, they can also teach you to control your attention and your impulses better.

Take plenty of sleep:

Sleep deprivation may increase adult ADHD symptoms, reducing the ability to cope with stress and remain concentrated during the daytime. Simple changes in daytime habits go a long way to ensuring nightly sleep is solid.

· Stop late-night caffeine.

· Exercise regularly and vigorously, but not within an hour of bedtime.

· Create a regular and quiet "bedtime" routine, including just before bed, taking a hot shower or bath.

· Stick to a regular schedule of sleep-wake even at weekends.

Eat healthily:

Although unhealthy eating habits do not cause ADHD, the symptoms may be exacerbated by a poor diet. Through making simple changes in what you eat and how you eat, you can experience significant reductions in levels of anxiety, hyperactivity, and stress.

· Eat tiny meals all day.

· Avoid as much as possible of the sugar and junk food.

· Make sure every meal includes healthy protein.

· Look for several portions of whole grains rich in fiber each day.

Practice mindfulness:

As well as reducing stress, regular meditation on mindfulness will help you better tolerate distractions, reduce impulsiveness, increase concentration, and provide more control over your emotions. Since the symptoms of hyperactivity can make meditation a challenge to some adults with ADHD, it can help to start slowly. Meditate for short periods and increase your meditation time slowly as you become more comfortable with the process— and are better able to keep focused. The goal is then to rely on these methods of mindfulness in your everyday life to keep you on track. Experiment with free or low-cost smartphone apps or guided meditations online.

4.6: Improve your communication skills in ADHD

Symptoms of ADHD can hinder communication. The following tips will help you converse more satisfyingly with your partner and other people.

Whenever possible, communicate face to face. Nonverbal signals like eye contact, tone of voice, and gestures convey much more than just words. To order to understand the meaning behind the words, you need to communicate with a person with your friend rather than by phone, text, or email.

Actively listen, and don't disturb. Make an effort to establish eye contact whilst the other person is talking. When you find your mind wandering, repeat their words internally, in order to follow the conversation. Make an effort not to interrupt.

Please ask questions. Rather than jumping into anything that's in your mind— or the many things in your mind — ask the other person a question. It is going to let them know that you pay attention to.

Demand a repeat. If your attention wanders, tell the other person and ask them to repeat what has just been said as soon as you realize it. When you allow the discussion to go too far while your mind is elsewhere, re-connecting will only become harder.

Manage feelings. If you are unable to discuss certain topics without flying off the handle or saying things that you regret later, consider meditating on mindfulness. As well as helping to reduce impulsiveness and increase concentration, regular meditation on mindfulness will give you greater control over your emotions and avoid emotional outbursts that can be so harmful to a relationship.

Chapter 5: Communication barrier and ADHD

ADHD treatment is never about focusing solely on attention or impulsiveness. ADHD reflects a deficiency in executive function, a collection of skills that involves concentration, management of impulses... and much more. Viewed as a self-regulation disorder, ADHD could have an effect on anything that needs planning and coordination, from sleep and eating habits to set up a long-term science project all the way to talking and listening in conversation.

Executive function serves as our' headmaster' in organizing our thought, behavior, and planning skills. It is responsible for processing all of the complex information that we encounter, from paying attention to the right voice in a classroom to coordinating answers in the middle of a fast-paced discussion. Comprehensive treatment for ADHD requires a broad view of its often-subtle effects on life, discussing its effect wherever it occurs. One of the dimensions of ADHD that are more often ignored is its direct impact on communication.

The Assessment and Statistical Manual of Mental Disorders (DSM) 5 is the official assessment manual for pediatric and mental health professionals. The new version, recently revised (though not published yet), divides communication into three components: speech-language, and pragmatics. Those skills are described as:

· Speech covers all that goes into sound production. Common speech problems include disorders of the articulation (unanticipated failure to make specific sounds), stuttering, and stammering.

· Language is what words mean and how we bring them together. This requires dialogue on vocabulary, grammar, and narration, along with corresponding sensitive language abilities. Specific disorders in this field under the present system are expressive language delays (such as using fewer words or sentences than anticipated) and receptive language delays (comprehending less than expected for age).

· Pragmatic language reflects all the nonverbal complexities that promote daily conversation and covers practically anything about the social side of communication. This includes all the unspoken facets of communication, such as reading faces and analysing voice tone, as well as responding to different situations (such as talking to a teacher versus a peer). Skills such as interpreting expressions, non-literal meetings (such as metaphor, irony, and sarcasm), and sensing the emotional meaning behind a facial expression transition, rely on an intuitive grasp of pragmatics.

5.1: Speech

Studies show that adults with ADHD are at risk of articulation disorders, which affect their ability to produce appropriate letter sounds for their age. Beyond that, fluency and voice quality often generally vary while speaking. Through these variations in expression, one study also found ADHD. Compared with peers with learning disabilities alone, individuals with ADHD displayed increased volume and pitch variation while speaking, along with specific patterns such as an increased number of vocal pauses.

Individuals with ADHD, when they try to organize their thoughts, create further verbal repetitions or word fillers, somewhat close to a stammer. This can lead to impatience and misunderstandings from others, especially children, since they do not usually have the same patience and experience as adults do. A classroom response maybe along the lines of, "It's an about story... um... a story... um... um... it's about... a kid who.... flies.... a.... kite... um."

5.2: Communication

People with ADHD process words even differently. They are at increased risk for major linguistic delays, for example. Even without specific delays, they are more likely to get off-topic when speaking due to distractibility and the related ADHD symptoms. I also often fail to find the right words to simply and linearly bring the ideas together in conversation. Grammatical errors as they compose sentences may also occur due to difficulties in planning, even when the underlying skills are intact in this area. All of these ADHD-related symptoms can impact the ability to communicate effectively, with or without actual language delays.

Within ADHD, listening comprehension can be specifically affected, particularly due to difficulties handling the speaking language or managing disruptive, noisy situations such as a party or a busy classroom. Also, even when a child has no apparent language delay, this is true; they have the capacity to understand, but due to ADHD, they lack information in speech as well as stories. They can lose track of conversational threads entirely or forget specifics while listening, and thus fail to capture crucial bits of information. These same discrepancies also surface as oppositional actions when a question seems to be deliberately overlooked rather than being addressed in the first place. Such trends often contribute to problems with reading comprehension frequently associated with ADHD.

It can become even more difficult for a child with ADHD in crowds or in a noisy environment to pay attention to the conversation thread. It is hard to be able to retain an emphasis on a single speaker and to switch between speakers. This has social implications, which causes some ADHD people to find it easier to get along one-on-one rather than in a group. Distracting classrooms can make it particularly difficult for a child with ADHD to participate when multiple events happen concurrently.

ADHD also often makes it difficult for a child to manage large conversational clumps all at once. While another 8-year-old may be able to handle listening at a clip of good understanding for as many as twelve terms, with ADHD, the limit could be seven or eight. Something bigger, and the knowledge starts dropping.

Such types of problems in the comprehension of spoken language are often incorrectly labeled as an' auditory processing disorder.' There is nothing wrong with the actual auditory pathway; the information gets in, but it is mismanaged by executive function. Once again, the brain manager is asleep on the job, jumbling the specifics of what is said.

5.3: Pragmatic

As noted above, the pragmatic language encompasses all the social mores associated with spoken language and nonverbal communication. Core ADHD symptoms all by themselves undermine this aspect of communication. For example, blurring responses, interrupting, talking unnecessarily, and speaking too loudly all violate common standards of communication. Individuals with ADHD also often make tangential conversational remarks or fail to coordinate their thoughts on the fly. Even for those with advanced vocabulary and age comprehension, these functional challenges may interfere with social success.

Such functional problems are similar to those found in an autistic person but not the same. The underlying issue in autism is that children do not intuitively grasp the social world — including pragmatic language delays. However, unlike those with ADHD, people with autism have an intrinsic developmental delay in a much wider range of social and communication skills.

For ADHD, it is most likely intact to be able to understand nonverbal language and social experiences as a whole. We recognize nonverbal communication for what it is, and understand basic communication rules such as' wait your turn to respond.' Due to distractibility, impulsiveness, or other impairments in the executive function, we can fail to follow those same rules at any given time, or even perceive social signals at all; many will meet criteria for a new DSM-5 category of' social (pragmatic) communication.

5.4: Actions speak louder than words

What can we do to deal with the personal and ADHD? Look for any potential linguistic delays. Intervene when necessary. And as adults, we adapt as much as possible to our own communication style.

Evaluate by direct monitoring for significant delays, and then implement necessary measures when indicated.

• Wait until you get the full attention of the person before making a request or starting a conversation; otherwise, the specifics are likely to be overlooked. Aid redirect their focus by using a brief marker, such as "Joseph, I've got a question for you." If it's effective, engage them verbally by gently touching their shoulder or a similar approach and then try to keep eye contact. The same approach (perhaps without the physical touch) helps people with ADHD in equal measure.

• Addressing realistic issues for individuals who struggle socially as behavioral therapy alone may not be enough, through collaborating with a therapist who is familiar with this communication dimension.

• Give ' extended conversational time,' allowing people who may struggle to get their thoughts together. Allow them enough time to settle down and coordinate their reactions.

• While speaking to someone with ADHD, often pause and break the language into shorter parts. Clearly announce, and use gesture language like counting bullet points on your fingers. If need be, rephrase or repeat yourself without judgment or condensation. Consider having kids restate what they got from what you said.

Chapter 6: Organizing home and office

Women are the main organizer of home they do know it how that have to manage their home well how to keep it organized, but for the women with ADHD it is quite difficult, and with that, if they are working women as well it just doubles the trouble for them.

Being focused and staying there is a real challenge for people living with ADHD. Some adults in both home and office may have difficulty with clutter and feel overwhelmed or stuck. Organizing yourself will benefit you in many ways, including:

· Increasing productivity.

· freeing time in search of things that reduce anxiety.

· serves as a positive role model for your children.

· To make more money efficiently.

· improving marriage, partnership, and other close relationships efficiently.

6.1: Strategies to get you motivated and keep you going

One of the hardest things to do is get going before you make a change. Positive improvements or incentives will help motivate you to organize yourself more. Pick a reward to offer yourself when you've done, before you start an organizing mission. Make sure you give yourself the award after you've completed the task.

Having a friend to help you, particularly if you need to declutter will make the job easier and go faster. Friends will help you get rid of things as they don't have the same sentimental attachment you have to them. You can also get mutual support from the online chat communities. Some have apps where you make specific commitments to organize a room and then walk away from your computer to organize for a while and then go back to their computers to support each other.

Using a timer and/or music can be of benefit. The timer may be programmed to go off if there are intervals of 15 minutes, with breathers in between. Many people find it helpful to put on a favorite playlist of songs, to start organizing, and to continue working until the playlist is over.

6.2: An effective strategy for getting organized

Learning a complex task is better done by breaking it down into smaller steps and approaching these steps one at a time. The organizing of a physical space can be divided into the following steps:

pick the spaces to be arranged and place them in order from the easiest to the most difficult start with the easiest time-space schedule to work on it, agree on the incentive or encouragement to promote the completion of each step to divide the space into work sections on one section at a time, sort, discard or reorganize each item

1. The very first step is to make a list of all the physical spaces that need to be organized, ranking the spaces from "easy to organize" to "most difficult to organize," using higher numbers for more complicated locations. You should post a copy of this document on a bulletin board or fridge door— somewhere you can always see it. First, start with the easiest space to maximize chances of success, then move on to the more challenging locations later.

Pick the space in your list that is easiest. Estimate how long you may be expected to arrange it. Choose a deadline to finish organizing this room. If the estimate is off, there may be additional time later to add. Split the estimated time into a number of short work sessions— between 30 and 60 minutes each. If you think in 30 to 60 minutes, you'd become irritated or depressed, shorten the session to 10 to 15 minutes and schedule more sessions. The goal is to start working for a short enough time without becoming depressed and exhausted, so you can achieve success. Schedule enough short planning sessions over the next few days or weeks to complete the task using a calendar, changing the estimate if appropriate. In the day planner, record the deadline and the time of the organization.

2. Divide the chosen space into parts or centers divide the area you work on into a grid, and focus on one part of the grid at a time. There are several ways of dividing space:

Quartering: visually divide the space into quarters, or mark it off using masking tape or string.

Divide the space into workable parts around the clock by breaking it like a clock. Stand at the room's doorway, render the spot at 12:00, and plan it first. Systematically work your way around the room, organizing the area at 1:00, 2:00, and 3:00, and so on until you get back to where you started. Tackle one or two "hours" of the clock during each of your planned planning sessions if doing the whole room this way is too much.

Zones: Organize the room parts according to location. Hold all the tools, materials, documents, and other things in that room zone for a given purpose. To organize your home office, for example, ask yourself what tasks might be performed in the workplace.

You agree that the following tasks will be carried out in the home office:

· Reading and responding to emails

· Surfing the Internet and making online transactions paying the bills,

· Making income taxes and completing other miscellaneous financial paperwork

· Writing technical papers and reading scientific journals

· Placing images and slides in folders and working on digital pictures on the computer.

The room could be organized into four zones.

Computer Zone — computer supplies on a desk, printer, modem, printer and computer, shopping catalogs, scientific journals and professional paper storage.

Camera Area — camera, video, lenses, camera accessories, negatives binders, and photo albums, and slides.

Financial Paperwork Zone — register financial reports, cabinets, accounts, extra receipts, bank books, and calculators.

Reading Area — a comfortable lounge chair with an overhanging lamp, a chairside table, and bookcases with books.

Draw a picture of the room on a piece of graph paper, study the current furniture configuration and decide how to rearrange the furniture to shape the four new zones. Only after preparing each zone and anticipating where the things will be placed in that zone can you move on to the next step — working on each area.

3. Working on each task Systematically gather everything you need to do the job (such as multiple boxes, plastic containers, garbage bags, masking tape, markers, pencil and paper, cleaning supplies, labels). Set your timer, or start the selected music. Start with three boxes and a bag of trash. Place any leftover food and empty food containers in the trash bag, mark the boxes "keep here," "Go somewhere else" or "not sure" Place any dirty dishes or silverware in the "go elsewhere" box to get back to the kitchen when finished.

Take in one item at a time. Decide which box belongs to the object, and decide if it is still useful to you. Put it in the garbage bag, if it is not. Place saved things either in the "keep here" box, if they belong to the section you're organizing now, or in the "go somewhere else" box if they belong to another section or room.

Do not take much time with every object. If you cannot decide to retain or discard the item quickly, place it in the "not sure" box. Continue going through items until all of the items in the segment are sorted, or the timer is gone, or the playlist is over. Then, pause for the day's job. Bring them out to the garbage. Remove the "go somewhere else" box and return those things to your "home." Don't worry that the homes may not yet be arranged for these items; just leave them in that section or space for now.

Keep the "not sure" box in the room until all of the things have been sorted. Then, seal the box with masking tape and close it. Write down on the outside of the box with a marker a potential date three to six months away. This is the day you reopen the box and check its contents. Label the date reopened in your day scheduler. Insert the box into a storage area. Take one of the following options while checking the products on the appointed day:

· If during the three- to six-month storage cycle, you have not had to search for the object in that package, then you don't need it. Put it into or give it away in the garbage.

· If you've hunted for the item, or now decide to keep it, find a home for it and place it there.

Felicitate yourself for your good work at the end of each organizing session, and give yourself the reward you have chosen.

4. Finish organizing the space repeat the steps to organize each section until the space is complete. Congratulate, and give yourself a big reward. Switch to the next item on the list of spaces to be arranged and follow the above steps. Continue to follow these measures until all the spaces are filled in the sequence.

6.3: Tips for staying organized

You want to keep them separated, after working very hard to organize the essential spaces in your life. Here are some ideas and tactics to help you keep the spaces decluttered.

Paperwork:

Four things to do with paper:

· Trash or recycle them.

· Refer it to someone else.

· Act on it now.

· Save or file it.

You can even reduce the need for paper handling in the future by removing your name from mailing lists. Catalog Choice is a service you can use to unsubscribe from various catalog mailing lists, and retailers have agreed to comply with those requests.

Another way to decrease paper is to use your camera, printer, or tablet to take pictures of the notes, letters, newspaper clippings, or other documents you want to save but don't need to have the originals of; save them to your computer and back up the files periodically. For easy access and scan, you can use the file folders to organize these images. Recycle that once you scan the file.

MAKE A TICKER FILING SYSTEM:

Your home or office is bombarded every day with the documents, notices, phone messages, newsletters, vouchers, bills, and mail you need to know about. The ticker system is a dated filing system that removes the piles, files, and lists that clutter your life. The system is made up of 43 directories, one marked each month (labeled January–December), and one marked each month's day (labeled 1–31).

Place the current month folder in front of folders numbered 1–31. Hold in plain sight these files (such as a folder standing on the desk or kitchen counter). Register those papers in the date folder you need to act on them. Do always remember to check the folders daily to make this system work.

At the end of each month, transfer the folder for the next month to the front and organize the items inside that folder into the corresponding regular numbered folders.

STORAGE STRATEGIES:

Try a few of the following techniques for neatly storing items and maintaining organization

· If you're not putting things away because you're scared, you're never going to find them, try storing them in clear containers. It will also save time being able to see inside the jar.

· To store things such as office supplies, shoes, clothing, tapes or DVDs, cleaning supplies, pantry items, baby care items, gloves, hats and scarves, and craft supplies, use over-the-door or hanging organizers with separated pouches in each room.

· Store tiny items with lids in boxes under the bed.

· To store extra sheets and blankets, or out of season clothing, buy a big trash can. Place it next to your bed, cover with a tablecloth over a floor and use it as a stand for the night.

The launch pad:

By setting up any table or small bookshelf by your front door for things you need when you leave your home, you can spend less time looking for stuff. Place a small basket or jar on the table to carry keys, glasses, and wallets. There you can also place briefcases and backpacks for the next morning.

CENTERS:

Establish centers that hold similar products and materials needed to accomplish a specific task. The products for each center, including bags, tackle boxes, buckets, and carts on wheels, can be stored in any suitable mobile container. This will save time because there will be one location for all the materials needed to complete a project. Make a list of the centers you are creating and the products in each center. Post the list to your newsletter so that you can quickly recall where those things are.

6.4: Eight ways to maintain a newly organized space

1. Handy box.

Keep a box or basket handy for out of place stuff as you clean up a room. If you come across things that are out of place, bring them in the bin. Upon completion of your room cleaning, take a few minutes to put these things in the proper room.

2. At the moment:

· Just close it as you pass an open cabinet.

· Pass a full wastebasket and empty it.

· Hang it up when you see a wardrobe item on the board.

· Bring them in the to-file box when you see some loose papers

3. Ten minutes pickup:

Spend 10 minutes on a quick pick-up each night. Bring a basket and go through the house, picking up things quickly and dropping them off where they belong. Better yet, include the whole family by making them clean up their room before bed each evening.

4. Quick clean up:

· Pick up the dropped stuff.

· Put away whatever you have used.

· Wipe up all the spill as soon as it happens.

5. Just for fifteen minutes:

· Set 15-minute timer.

· Those 15 minutes concentrate your attention on one thing.

· Decide if you can keep going for another 15 minutes when the timer goes off.

· Set the timer again for the next 15 minutes if you can.

· If you can't, just stop and do the same later in the day or the next, until the project you're trying to finish is done

It might seem like a short time, but it will soon make a difference. You can always see and experience what these 15 minutes have achieved.

6. Subtract before you add:

Consider yourself a rule- "Subtract always before you add!" If you subtract one (such as no new books or magazines if you read or give away unread books or magazines), you will not add (purchase) a new object.

7. Put in place:

Every time there are a few minutes to spare, put away five or ten items that are not in their right place. These could be toys that the children left behind, letters that need to be filed away, or socks to be put in the drawer.

8. Toss box:

Keep a box or bag inside a storage area to store donated items. As you notice an item you don't want or use, take it to the donate box straight away. Don't allow unwanted or unused items to take up valuable space awaiting a regular dig-out. Place small objects in the garbage, and larger items in a trash pick-up day storage area.

Get Started:

After reading those suggestions, some readers will be able to start organizing. Others might find they need a mentor, professional organizer, or therapist's support to get started. Don't quit or give up when you need help. It took a lifetime to get to the state of disorganization that you were living in; it will take time to fix it. The secret to the beginning.

Chapter 7: ADHD women and marriage

Marriage has a great impact on women's lives, and as per the tradition of the world we are living it is a women's duty to take care of martial life and women suffering from ADHD often find it difficult to deal with it because, in your closest relationships, ADHD will trigger misunderstandings, tensions, and anger. There are, however, ways of creating a healthier and happier relationship.

The numbers are frightening, and sometimes you may not think it's possible to work with ADHD in the mix for a family. You compete too much. Your home is something of a mess. They can't find their keys. When you recall that you have them, you're late for appointments. The payments will be late. You say things during important conversations without thought, or block them out. Everything is in turmoil. And yet, people with ADHD are fully capable of fulfilling and happy relationships.

Both relationships have their ups and downs, but the partnership is significantly more challenging if one or both partners have ADHD. Two men, two lives intertwined, under one roof every day and ADHD. It is complicated, and it is challenging, it is beautiful, it's not impossible.

Marriage is something of a cord. The entangled threads can be either solid or frayed. The rope remains strong and supportive as you mutually touch and ascend upwards. But the threads can get twisted and frayed with too much stress, the rope weakens, and gradually your relationship begins to break apart.

The good news is you always play an active part in your marriage. You can choose your position, how you interact, and the behaviors that can either reinforce your bond or weaken it. If you're ready and willing to reinforce the cord that binds you and your partner together, you'll bring back the dry, cozy feeling you had when you first met.

When did you meet? Remember the sparks that flew between you when you looked into each other's eyes? There was something about this person that made you want to spend the rest of your life together. The feeling can be brought back again. In reality, if you choose to make an effort, it can be even better than that - a stronger, more mature, and deeper connection.

Relationships flourish when both spouses behave lovingly towards each other, willing to make a thorough effort and committed to working on their own.

7.1: How does ADHD or ADD affect relationships?

While the distractibility, disorganization, and impulsivity of attention deficit hyperactivity disorder (ADHD or ADD) may cause problems in many areas of adult life, these symptoms may be especially damaging when it comes to your closest relationships. This is especially true if there has never been a proper diagnosis or treatment of ADHD symptoms.

If you're the ADHD person, you may feel like you're being constantly criticized, nagged, and micro-managed. No matter what you do, it seems like nothing pleases your spouse or partner. As an adult, you don't feel respected, and you find yourself avoiding your partner or doing anything you need to get them off your back. You wish that your significant other might just relax a bit and stop trying to control every aspect of your life. You wonder what happened to that person with whom you fell in love.

If you're in a relationship with someone who's getting ADHD, you may feel lonely, neglected, and hated. You're sick of being the only responsible party in the relationship and taking care of everything on your own. You do not feel like you can rely on your friend. We never seem to follow through on promises, and you are continually forced to issue reminders and requests or simply do it yourself. Sometimes it seems like it just doesn't care about your significant other.

It is clear to see how emotions on both sides will lead to the relationship's destructive cycle. The non-ADHD partner cries, nags, and becomes more resentful while the ADHD partner becomes protective and pulls away, feeling humiliated and confused. No-one is happy at the end. But this should not be the way it is. Through learning about the role ADHD plays in your relationship and how both of you can choose more positive and productive ways to respond to challenges and connect with each other, you can create a stronger, happier partnership. You will add greater understanding to your relationship with these approaches, and bring you closer together.

7.2: Understanding the role of ADHD in adult relationships

The improvement of your relationship starts with an understanding of the role ADHD plays. Once you can identify how the ADHD symptoms influence your interactions as a couple, you can learn better ways to respond. This means learning how to handle the symptoms of an ADHD partner. This means to the non-ADHD partner learning how to react to conflicts in ways that empower and inspire the partner.

Symptoms of ADHD which can cause:

Trouble paying attention to relationship problems. If you have ADHD, during interactions, you might zone out, which could make your partner feel neglected and devalued. You may also miss important information or consent to something that you later don't recall, which can be irritating to your loved one.

Forgetting. Even if someone with ADHD is paying attention, they might later forget what was promised or spoken about. When it's the birthday of your spouse or the formula you said you'd pick up, your partner may start feeling like you don't care or you're unreliable.

Bad skills in management. This can contribute to both difficulties in completing tasks and general chaos in the household. Partners may feel like they're cleaning up a disproportionate amount of family duties after the person with ADHD.

Impulsion. If you have ADHD, without thinking, you may blur things out, which can cause hurt. Such impulsiveness can also lead to careless and even reckless behavior (for example, making a big purchase which is not in the budget, leading to fights over finances).

Outbursts of emotion. Most people living with ADHD have difficulty moderating their emotions. You can quickly lose your temper and have difficulty peacefully discussing issues. Your partner may feel like they're going on eggshells to prevent blow-ups.

7.3: Put yourself in your partner's shoes

Learning to see things from your partner's perspective is the first step in turning your relationship around. If you've been together for a long time, or have had the same struggles over and over again, you may think you already understand where your partner comes from. But don't underestimate the simplicity of misinterpreting the actions and intentions of your partner. You and your partner are different from what you think— especially if one of you only has ADHD. And just because you've heard it all before, that doesn't mean you've really gotten into what your partner says. If emotions run high, as they normally do around issues relating to ADHD, it is particularly difficult to maintain objectivity and perspective.

The easiest way of putting yourself in the shoes of your friend is to inquire, and then just listen. If you're not already angry, find a time to sit down and chat. Let your partner clarify how they feel to justify or defend themselves from you without interruption. Read back the main points you've heard them say when your partner is done, and ask if you understood correctly. You might want to write down the details, so you can think about them later. It's your turn when your partner is finished. Ask them to do the same for you, listen with fresh ears and an open mind, really.

7.4: Tips for increasing understanding in your relationship

Research ADHD right up. The more you both learn about ADHD and its symptoms, the easier it'll be to see how it affects your relationship. You can notice a light bulb is turning on. So many of your problems end up being important as a couple! Recalling that a brain with ADHD is hardwired differently than an ADHD-free brain can help the non-ADHD partner take symptoms less personally. For the ADHD parent, realizing what's behind some of your actions can be a comfort–and recognizing there are steps you can take to control your symptoms.

Recognize the impact your conduct has on your partner. It's important to recognize how your unresolved symptoms affect your partner if you're the one with ADHD. If you're the parent outside of ADHD, remember how the nagging and criticism makes your spouse feel. Don't dismiss or disregard your partner's complaints, because you don't like how they bring them up or react to you.

Separate your partner from any of their signs or behaviors. Instead of labeling your partner "irresponsible," recognize their forgetfulness as symptoms of ADHD and lack of follow-throughs. Remember, character traits are not symptoms. The same goes for the parent who is not ADHD too. Recognize that nagging usually results from anger and anxious feelings, not because your partner is an unsympathetic harpy.

7.5: How the partner of with ADHD feels

Different. The brain is often running, so people with ADHD view the world in a way other people don't understand or respond easily to.

They are overwhelmed by the constant stress induced by signs of ADHD, whether unconsciously or overtly. It takes much more work to keep the daily life under control than others realize. Even if it's not always apparent, ADHD will make someone feel like they are trying to keep their head above water.

Subordinate to married couples. Their spouses spend a considerable amount of time correcting or running the show. The corrections make them feel inept, and they often lead to a dysfunctional parent-child. Men may define such experiences as emasculating them.

Shamed. Fucked. We also hide a great deal of guilt, often making up for bluster or withdrawal.

Unloved and unacceptable. Constant reminders from spouses, bosses, and others that they are supposed to "change," reinforce their unlikeness as it is.

Fear of failure again. With their relationships weakening, the potential for retribution for failure is growing. But its contradictions arising from ADHD mean that at some stage, this partner will struggle. Anticipating failure leads to an unwillingness to try.

Longing for recognition. One of those with ADHD's greatest emotional needs is to be loved just as they are, despite imperfections.

7.6: How the partner with non-ADHD feels

Unwanted or hated. The lack of focus is perceived as not a distraction but a lack of interest. One of the most common dreams is to be "confirmed," and to obtain the love that this means from one's spouse.

Angry and frustrated, mentally. Anger and resentment permeate a lot of spousal interactions with ADHD. The rage is sometimes conveyed as a disconnection. Some non-ADHD spouses try to block their feelings by bottling them up inside, in an effort to control angry interactions.

Extremely stressed out. Non-ADHD partners also bear the overwhelming share of family responsibilities and can never let down their guard. At any time, life could fall apart because of the incoherence of the ADHD spouse.

Ignored, and he was offended. It doesn't make sense to a non-ADHD spouse that the ADHD spouse doesn't rely on the experience and advice of the non-ADHD partner more often when what needs to be done is "simple."

Drained and drained. The non-ADHD partner has too many obligations, and there seems to be a little amount of effort to repair the relationship.

Frowned. A non-ADHD partner may feel like the same issues come up again and again (a sort of boomerang effect).

7.7: Take responsibility for your role

Once you've put yourself in the shoes of your partner, it's time to take responsibility for your role in the partnership. Once you become conscious of your own contributions to the issues you have as a couple, improvement begins. This also refers to the Non-ADHD spouse.

While the symptoms of the ADHD spouse can cause a problem, it is not the symptoms alone that fault the relationship problem. The manner in which the non-ADHD spouse reacts to the embarrassing symptom can either open the door to collaboration and reconciliation or trigger misunderstandings and hurt feelings. If you are the one with ADHD, then you are also responsible for how you react to the issues of your family. Your response can either support and understand your significant other or dismiss and ignore them.

Break free of the parent-child dynamic:

Most couples feel stuck in an unsatisfying kind of partnership between parent and child, with the non-ADHD partner in the role of the parent and the partner with ADHD in the role of the child. It often begins when the ADHD partner fails to carry out tasks such as forgetting to pay the cable bill, leaving clean laundry in a pile on the bed, or leaving the children stranded after promising to pick them up. The non-ADHD parent is gradually assuming responsibility for the households.

The more that relationship is lopsided, the more resentful they become. It's getting harder to recognize the positive qualities and achievements of the ADHD partner. The ADHD parent, of course, feels this. We begin to feel that there is no point in even trying, and ignore the non-ADHD partner as being manipulative and unpleasant. So, what are you going to do to break that pattern?

Tips for the non-ADHD partner:

· You can't control your partner, but you can keep your own actions under control. Put the verbal attacks and nagging to an immediate stop. Neither's getting results.

· Encourage your partner to make progress and recognize achievements and efforts.

· Try to focus, where possible, on the motives of your partner, rather than what they actually do. For example, they can lose focus while listening to you, but that doesn't mean they don't care about what you've got to say.

· Stop trying to have your partner, "dad." This destroys your friendship and demotivates your partner.

Tips for the partner with ADHD:

·   Recognize the interference your ADHD symptoms have with your relationship. It is not just a case of being unreasonable to your partner.

· Consider choices for the diagnosis. Your companion will ease as you learn to manage your symptoms and become more consistent.

· If strong emotions disrupt interactions with your partner, decide in advance that you need to take some time out to calm down and refocus before you continue.

· Find ways to spoil your husband. If your partner feels that you matter about them— even in small ways — they may feel less like their parent.

7.8: Stop fighting and start communicating

As you have already learned, when ADHD is in the mix, contact also breaks down between partners. One partner feels heavy-handed. The other one feels aggressed. They end up fighting each other instead of tackling the problem.

Do what you can to defuse emotional uncertainty, to improve communication. Take time to cool off before discussing a matter if necessary. Listen closely to your friend when you have the talk. Ask yourself exactly what you are arguing about. Which is the deeper problem?

For example, it is an hour late for a couple to fight over dinner. The husband, who has no ADHD, is more concerned about his empty stomach than his. He feels frustrated with the lack of commitment and affection from his wife (I'm working hard to provide for her! Why don't I ever get any TLC? If she cared for me, she would make more effort!). The wife of ADHD feels overwhelmed and unfairly judged (I've got so much to look after around the house. It's hard for me to keep up with everything, and I've lost track of time. How does that make me a bad wife?).

When you identify the real issue, the problem can be solved much more quickly. In this example, if he realized his wife's chronic lateness and disorganization is not personal, the husband would be less upset. It is an unresolved sign of

ADHD. On her part, once the wife knows that her husband's feeling loved and appreciated by a timely meal, she will be more motivated to make it happen.

Don't lock the emotions up. Fess your emotions, no matter how ugly that may be. Get them out into the open, where you can work as a couple with them.

You are not a teacher of minds. Don't make any assumptions about the motives of your partner. Evite the pit "if my wife really loved me...." If your partner is doing something that upsets you, fix it straight away rather than stewing quietly.

Know what you're doing and how you're doing it. Avoid provocative terms and questions put on the defensive by your partner ("Why can't you ever do what you said you'd do?" or "How many times do I have to remind you?").

Tackle the situation with irony. Learn to laugh about inevitable miscommunications and miscomprehensions. Laughter relieves stress and unites you together.

7.9: Do the teamwork

Just because one of the partners has ADHD doesn't mean that you can't have a balanced relationship that fulfills one another. The secret is the ability to work as a team together. A healthy relationship involves giving and taking, with both parties becoming fully involved in the partnership and looking for ways to support one another.

Take some time to determine what you're good at and which things are most daunting to you on both sides. If your partner is strong in an environment where you are weak, they might be able to take on that responsibility, and vice versa. It should feel a level playing field. When both of you are poor in a given area, imagine how to get support from outside. For example, if you're not good at finance, you might be able to hire a bookkeeper or research money management apps that makes it easier to budget.

Divide and hold on to duties. While managing the kids and cooking, the non-ADHD partner may be more suited to handling bills and doing the errands.

Schedule the sit-downs weekly. Meet as a couple once a week to tackle issues and assess the progress you have achieved.

Evaluate the labor division. Make a list of duties and obligations and rebalance the workload if one of you shoulder the bulk of the bill.

Delegate and outsource. Automate. You do not do everything yourself and your friend. If you have kids delegate tasks to them, you may also consider hiring a cleaning service, signing up for delivery of foodstuffs, or setting up automated bill payments.

If required, divide up individual tasks. If the ADHD partner has trouble completing tasks, the non-ADHD partner may need to step in as the "closer." Plan in your agreement for this to prevent resentment.

Create a practical plan:

If you have ADHD, you are probably not very good at setting up or managing processes. But that doesn't mean that once it's in place, you cannot obey a strategy. This is an environment where a non-ADHD friend can provide invaluable support. We will help you set up a system and schedule that you can count on to help you keep up with your obligations.

Start by analysing the most common things you struggle with, like chores or chronic lateness. Then think about practical things to fix. It might be a big wall calendar with check boxes next to the daily tasks of each individual forgotten chores. You could set up a calendar on your smartphone for chronic lateness, complete with timers to remind you of coming events.

7.10: Helping your partner with ADHD

Work out a routine. The added framework would benefit your partner. Timing the tasks, you both need to do and accept fixed food, workout, and sleep times.

Set up alerts outside. This can be in the form of a dry erase board, sticky notes on your phone, or a to-dodo list.

Command fear. People with ADHD have difficulty getting organized and staying organized, but clutter adds to the feeling their lives are out of control. Help your partner set up a clutter control and structured stay program.

Demand a repeat request from the ADHD parent. Have your friend explain what you agreed to6 avoid misunderstandings.

7.11: Ways to have happy marriage

Everyone has a dark side, and all you need is love to feel down, right? Incorrect. If you or your partner has ADHD, follow these rules to promote communication, build confidence, and reciprocate support.

Whatever the adult attention deficit disorder (ADHD or ADD), it's easy to fall in love. A surge of biochemical euphoria comes with "new love." Those of us with ADHD frequently concentrate on sex, not only for the sake of romance but also to enhance those neurotransmitters (dopamine), generating pleasure that is in short supply throughout our brains. Highly charged emotions do not form part of enduring love. These are just feelings — strong and wonderful feelings — but you need a lot more to finish off an ADHD relationship.

Relationships are hard, and when we accept that fact, we're dealing with reality, not with the illusion that "love is all you need." I don't believe it. To make up for your weaknesses and save your relationship, you need coping skills. What tools should you have in your toolbox for the relationship? Glad you have asked.

Games. But do your best with your positive side to make decisions, and "run your life."

1. Manage Symptoms.

You and your partner will consider your condition as their own. Treat ADHD responsibly with behavioral therapy and/or appropriate drugs to manage symptoms, increase dopamine, and help the brain function as it should. You should see a reduction in ADHD symptoms when you do all that— like the inability to focus while your partner is talking to you or perform tasks like paying bills on time.

Not being heard is a big complaint from those in close relationships with ADHD partners. Listening to others is difficult for many who have ADHD. Practice this exercise to improve your listening skills: sit down with your partner and let him talk for five minutes— or longer, if you can. Make eye contact and lean into him, even if not every word is absorbed.

After five minutes of listening, sum up what you've heard. You might tell, "Wow, it sounds like you've had a hectic day: the awful walk, the dreadful meeting. You've got to stop at the gym on the way home, at least. "Do something you want to do after the trade. Ask, "When you're home now, will you bother to watch Robbie while I'm running?" Probably your partner will be shocked and pleased you've been listening to him for five minutes.

2. Commit to Commitment

ADHD's key symptoms — impulsiveness and the need for constant stimulation — can strengthen relationships, as well as disrupt them. Adventurous sexual activities are particularly stimulating because people with ADHD are restless and easily bored. Attraction to the new and the special will make it hard to remain monogamous. That's why sticking to the notion of "relationship" is vital— even more so than being your partner.

I met a 93-year-old woman who spent more than 70 years marrying the same man. She told me that, in their years together, they had good times and bad times, and that she had never considered divorce once, although she joked that she had considered murder once or twice. She knew that to make the relationship work, she had to be more committed to the institution of marriage than to her husband. There were times when the couple didn't feel dedicated to each other, but they got through their commitment to their marriage.

3. Use Laughter Therapy

Learn to laugh at yourself (not your partner) and take your issues a little easier. ADHD sometimes causes us to do and say some quite unusual things.

Rather than being hurt or angry by unintentional words and deeds, see them for what they are: the manifestations of a disease that you try to manage. A good laugh helps you advance in the relationship. I know how tough that can be. It's easy to be defensive because we've had to justify our actions for years — when we were behaving impulsively or glossing over specifics due to lack of focus. Drop the defensiveness and then let go.

4. Forgive and Forget

It's easy to point your finger at the other person and blame her for the relationship problems. Yet tango needs two. Instead of dwelling on what our spouse does wrong, we grow spiritually as we accept the issues we may be causing. When I recognize my own deficiencies — identify them, work to change them, and forgive myself for not being perfect— it's easier to accept my partner and forgive her deficiencies.

Another sentence that sums up this idea of forgiving-and-forgetting is: "At that moment, I did the best I could do. If I could have done better, I'd have. "It takes the sting from a bad experience and encourages you and your partner to speak to each other civilly. It's no longer about "doing it again" one of you, it's about being human and making mistakes—something you can forgive.

5. Seek Professional Help

Many married couples with one or more spouses diagnosed with ADHD plan to get married "until death do us part." But as the challenges of living together set in, little problems go unnoticed and become bigger problems that seem insurmountable.

One of the common mistakes that unhappy couples make is to wait too long for their relationship to get professional help. By the time they get to the therapist's office, they've already thrown into the towel, finding only a way to validate their suffering and justify their divorce decision. Don't wait too long for some help. A licensed marriage therapist and family therapist will teach communication skills and conflict resolution.

More ADHD Relationship Tools:

- When you first fell in love, remember to keep doing the fun things you did together.
- Make a rule: Just one insane person at a time in the house. You have to keep cool and collected while your friend is flipping out.
- Each week, go on a date.
- Have respect for one another. Know the quirks of loving one another.
- Allow no concerns about who's right. The goal is to advance— not remain trapped in an argument. Having

a relationship that is mutually satisfying is more important than being right all the time.

Chapter 8: Succeeding in the workplace

Some adult females with ADHD have jobs that are very productive. But for others, ADHD's symptoms can present a variety of challenges, including poor communication skills, distractibility, procrastination, and complex project management difficulties. Here are some of the challenges and strategies for getting through them.

Challenge: Distractibility:

There are two forms of disturbances, external and internal, that may affect adults working with ADHD. External involve items such as sounds or movement in the surrounding environment while internal disturbances, such as daydreams, occur internally.

Suggestion: Headphones with noise cancelation can help minimize ambient noises. If you have an office, consider closing your door to prevent disturbance on the part of your officers. Restrict your social media exposure when you need to get things done. To-dodo lists will help you stay up to the task and battle your daydreaming.

Challenge: Impulsivity:

When frustrated, adults with ADHD may be fighting impulsivity and excessive temper.

Suggestions: Self-talking, collaborating with a mentor, receiving consistent and positive input, cultivating empathy, and developing coping mechanisms will help adults learn how to recognize their causes and communicate their emotions in appropriate ways.

Challenge: Hyperactivity:

ADHD adults often have trouble sitting still and may get fidget.

Suggestions: Consider jobs that allow movement or require a great deal of physical activity such as sales, teaching, or exercise trainers. For those in more sedentary jobs, take occasional breaks, take notes at meetings, and walkabout. You can also bring your lunch, so you don't have to spend time buying it, and instead, you can use your break to workout.

Challenge: Poor Memory.

Failure to recall deadlines and details of a project can have a negative effect on job performance.

Suggestions: Use tape recording tools to record data, write checklists for complicated tasks, or use reminders for announcements such as sticky notes or memory triggers.

Challenge: Boredom-block outs.

Some adults with ADHD get more easily bored at work, especially when doing detailed paperwork and routine tasks, from a need for simulation.

Suggestions: To avoid boredom, set a timer to stay on task, split long tasks into shorter ones, take breaks to get up and walk around, or find a job with responsibilities that stimulate and minimize routine tasks.

Challenge: Time Management.

People with ADHD have a more difficult time monitoring time than people who don't. We may not know just how long a job takes.

Suggestions: Split bigger projects into smaller pieces with individual due dates to prevent a waste of time. Award yourself for achieving every goal, using alarms, buzzers, etc. to recall meets and other activities.

Challenge: Procrastination.

To people with ADHD, putting things off can seem like second nature.

Suggestions: Split assignments into small parts, enlist the help of your boss in setting deadlines to tasks, if possible, or collaborate with a co-worker who handles time well.

Challenge: Paperwork/Details.

The inability to find important papers, send in reports and timesheets, and maintain a filling schedule will seriously hinder one's ability to get timely work done.

Suggestions: Build a filing system that works for you or ask an administrative assistant to manage comprehensive paperwork and delete papers that you don't use daily.

Challenge: Interpersonal/Social Skills.

Individuals with ADHD may involuntarily offend colleagues by repeatedly interrupting, talking too much, being too blunt, or not listening well.

Suggestions: Ask for input from others, learn to read social cues, collaborate with a mentor, or search for a place where you can be your own boss.

Challenge: Difficulty in managing long-term projects.

Managing complex or long-term tasks may be the most challenging organizational task for adults with ADHD due to time management issues, managing resources, monitoring progress, and communicating achievements.

Suggestions: To make long-term projects easier to manage, divide them into smaller parts; shorten the time required on the project to make better use of' sprinting skills;' collaborate with a co-worker; or if you can't handle long-term projects at all, look for work that needs only short-term tasks.

Chapter 9: ADHD and social life

The behavior of individuals with ADHD is often seen as impulsive, disorganized, aggressive, overly sensitive, intense, emotional, or disruptive. In their social environment, their social interactions with others— parents, siblings, teachers, friends, co-workers, spouses / partners — are often filled with misunderstanding and miscommunication.

Those with ADHD have a diminished ability to self-regulate their behavior and reactions towards others. That can lead to overly strained and unstable relationships.

The subjects in this segment deal with some of the common relationship issues faced by women with ADHD and others in their lives.

Social skills in women with ADHD.

Individuals with ADHD also encounter social difficulties as a result of their inattention, impulsiveness and hyperactivity, social rejection, and interpersonal relationship issues. These negative interpersonal outcomes cause both mental pain and suffering. These also appear to help improve co-morbid mood disorders and anxiety disorders.

Since very little research on social skills in adults with ADHD has been written, the recommendations in this sheet are based primarily on sound clinical practices and upward extrapolations from research on social skills for children and ADHD.

9.1: Overall impact on social interaction

The reasons why people with ADHD sometimes struggle in social situations are not difficult to comprehend. One of the most important aspects of a child's development is to actively connect with peers and significant adults, but 50 to 60 percent of children with ADHD have trouble with peer relationships.

More than 25 percent of Americans feel persistent loneliness. One can only guess that adults with ADHD are much higher in percentage.

An individual has to be attentive, responsible, and able to control impulsive behaviors to interact effectively with others. Adults with ADHD are often inattentional and forgetful, and usually lack control of impulses. Since ADHD is an "invisible disability," frequently unacknowledged by those who may not be familiar with the disease, other factors are often linked to socially inappropriate actions arising from ADHD symptoms. That is, people also view these behaviors and the individual who conducts them as rude, self-centered, reckless, lazy, mischievous, and a host of other negative attributes of personality. With time, these misleading labels lead to the person with ADHD being socially rejected. Social rejection creates emotional pain in the lives of many of the children and adults who have ADHD, and throughout their life, may create havoc and lower self-esteem. The improper social behavior in relationships and marriages will annoy the partner or spouse without ADHD who may ultimately "blackout" and give up on the relationship or marriage.

Educating people with ADHD, their significant ones, and their families about ADHD and the ways it affects social skills and behavioral habits will help relieve much of the tension and blame. At the same time, women with ADHD need to learn strategies to become as proficient in the field of social skills as possible. Through proper evaluation, care, and education, individuals through ADHD may learn to successfully communicate with others in a way that improves their social life.

9.2: ADHD and the acquisition of social skills

In general, social skills are learned by indirect learning: watching people, observing others ' behavior, practicing, and getting feedback. Some people begin this process early in their infancy. Social skills are learned and developed by "playing grown-up" and other behaviors of childhood. Observation and peer feedback sharpen the finer points of social interactions.

These specifics are often overlooked by children with ADHD. We can pick up bits and pieces of what's right, but we lack a general view of social standards. Sadly, they frequently know that "something" is lacking as adults but are never quite sure what this "something" maybe.

Public acceptance can be seen as a continuum of ups and downs. Individuals with adequate social skills are rewarded with greater acceptance from those they communicate with and are motivated to learn even better social skills. The spiral also goes down towards those with ADHD. A lack of social skills leads to peer rejection, which then restricts social skills learning opportunities, leading to more rejection, and so on. Social punishment involves dismissal, avoidance, and other, less overt ways of expressing disapproval of one another.

It's important to note that people sometimes don't let the offending person know about the extent of the infringement. It is often considered socially unacceptable to point out that a mistake in social skills is being made. Therefore, people are often left alone to try to improve their social skills without understanding exactly what areas need to be changed.

9.3: Specific ADHD symptoms and social skills

INATTENTION:

Tips for identifying subtext:

· Look for clues to help you decode the subtext within your context. Be mindful of possible alternatives. Be cautious.

· Be mindful of body language, voice tone, actions, or somebody's eyes look to help understand what they're saying.

· To spot the subtext better, look at a person's choice of words. ("I'd love to go" probably means yes. "If you want to" probably doesn't mean it, but I'm going to do it.) Acts speak louder than words. If somebody's words say one thing, but their actions reveal another, it would be wise to take into account that their actions might reveal their feelings.

· Find out a guide to help you with this language of hiding. Compare your conception of reality with your understanding of reality. If there's a difference, you may want to try understanding the other person and see what's happening, particularly if you normally get it wrong.

· Know how to interpret friendly attitudes. Sometimes, politeness disguises real feelings.

· Be vigilant about what others do. Look around for clues on proper behavior, clothing, seating, parking, and the like.

· A momentary lapse of attention could result in a social interaction in which the person with ADHD loses important information. If a simple phrase like "Let's meet at noon at the park," actually becomes "Let's meet at noon," then the listener with ADHD loses the crucial information about the meeting's place. When the listener asks where will be the meeting will take place, the speaker may become frustrated or annoyed, believing that the listener was deliberately not paying attention and did not value what they had to say. Or worse still, the adult with ADHD goes to the wrong location, causing the partner frustration and even rage. Sadly, sometimes neither the speaker nor the audience knows that until it's too late, important information was missing.

For many women with ADHD, a related social skills challenge includes lacking the subtle nuances of communication. Those with ADHD will often fail to "read between the lines" or grasp subtext. It is sufficiently difficult for most people to attend to the conversation text without having to be aware of the subtext and what the person really means. Sadly, what's said is often not really what's said.

IMPULSIVITY:

Impulsivity has a negative impact on social relationships, as others may attribute impulsive words or actions to a lack of care or consideration for others. Failure to stop and reflect often has catastrophic social consequences at first. Impulsivity in speech may appear as unfiltered thinking, without self-editing what is about to be said. Opinions and ideas are conveyed in their raw form, without the normal veneer that is socially appropriate for most people. Breakdowns are common.

Impulsive acts can also cause difficulties as individuals with ADHD can act through their behavior before thinking. Taking decisions based on a philosophy of "in the moment" also leads to poor decision-making. Those with ADHD often find that something more inviting lures them off the task. Impulsive acts can include taking careless risks, failing to research or plan for school-or work-related projects, doing business, leaving jobs, making moving decisions, financial overspending, and even aggressive actions like hitting others or throwing items.

Rapid, too much speech can also be a sign of impulsiveness. An individual's speaking with ADHD quick-fire leaves little room for others who might want to engage in the conversation. Monologues leave many with ADHD without fulfilling relationships or needing details, rather than dialogues.

Hyperactivity:

The ability to engage in leisure activities is often limited by physical hyper activeness. Others may interpret the failure to sit still and concentrate on concerts, religious ceremonies, educational events, or even leisure vacations and the like as a lack of care or concern on the part of the person with ADHD. Furthermore, difficulties that look attentive leave others feeling unattended.

9.4: Social skills assessment

Interviews and self-report questionnaires are the primary tools used in individuals with ADHD to evaluate social skill deficiencies and interpersonal interaction issues. During a medical examination of ADHD, a mental health professional must carefully examine the adult's social interactions. When using questionnaires, it is important to include on a comparable version of the questionnaire both an individual's self-report of ADHD and reports from partners, significant others, and friends. The questionnaire can include the following articles:

Difficulty paying attention when spoken to, missing pieces of information. Appears to ignore others.

Difficulty taking turns in conversation (tendency to interrupt frequently) Difficulty pursuing tasks and/or responsibilities.

Failure to use proper ways.

Missed social indications.

Disorganized lifestyle Sharing information that is inappropriate.

Being distracted by sounds or noises.

Become frustrated or overwhelmed.

Shutting down disorganized or dispersed thoughts.

Rambling or straying off topic during conversations.

9.5: Ways to Master Social Skills

Social skills can often be significantly improved when there is an awareness of social skills as well as the areas that need to be changed. Reading books like What Does Anyone Know That I Don't Know, ADD and Love, or You, Your Marriage & ADD can provide some of that information.

Attitude: Attitude. Individuals with ADHD should have a positive attitude and be open to improving their social skills.

It is also important to be open and appreciative of other people giving input.

Targets. Adults with ADHD might want to pick and focus on one target at a time, based on self-assessment and others ' evaluations. Tackling the areas of expertise one at a time allows the person to master each skill before moving on to the next.

The resounding. Those who struggle with missing pieces of information during conversation due to concentration problems that benefit from developing a system of reviewing what they heard with others. "I have heard you say this. Had I got it right is there more "Or a person with ADHD may ask others to check with them after they have provided important information. "Just tell me what you heard me say." That way, it's possible to avoid social mistakes due to inattention.

Keep others out. Adults suffering from ADHD will learn a lot by watching others do what they need to do. They may want to try selecting models to help them grow in this area, both at work and in their personal lives. The TV can also provide role models.

Playing position. Practicing the skills, they need with others is a good way for people with ADHD to get input and develop their social skills as a result.

Visualization. Visualization can be used to gain additional experience and boost one's capacity in other environments to apply the skill. Those who need social skills practice can decide what they want to do and rehearse it in their minds, imagining that they will actually use the skills in the setting they will be in with the people they will actually interact with. To further "overlearn" the ability, they should practice this as many times as possible. In this way, they will gain experience in the "real" world, which will greatly increase their prospect of success.

Good luck. Adults with ADHD may use reminders to stay focused on specific social ability objectives. The prompts can be visual (an index card), or verbal (someone telling them to be quiet), physical (a vibrating watch set every 4 minutes reminding them to be quiet), or a gesture (someone rubbing their heads) to help them recall working on their social skills.

Increase "likelihood." People maintain relationships based on how well those relationships meet their needs, according to social exchange theory. Individuals are not necessarily "social accountants," but individuals weigh the costs and benefits of being in relationships on some point. Many with ADHD are known to be "high maintenance," so seeing what they can bring to relationships to help balance the equation is beneficial. Investigators have found the following attributes to be very likable: genuine, honest, compassionate, respectful, fair, trustworthy, knowledgeable, professional, conscientious, considerate, efficient, dry, caring, polite, pleasant, unselfish, humorous, responsible, cheerful and trustful. The creation or enhancement of any of the features of likeability will boost one's social standing.

Although ADHD often poses unique challenges to social relationships, it offers information and resources to help people with ADHD develop their social skills. Most of this information is based on sound clinical practice and research on social skills and ADHD in children and adolescents; more research on social skills and ADHD in adults is a great necessity. Seek help through reading, counseling, or coaching, and build and maintain social connections above all else.

9.6: Friendship and ADHD women

It is difficult for women with ADHD to hang on to friendships. They feel squeezed by the expectations of society that they feel destined to miss. Understanding the brain of ADHD and the impact it has on social skills can reduce the shame and increase opportunities for meaningful connection.

Friendship Challenges for Adult Women with ADHD

Peer acceptance is a potent measure of women's self-worth. The strength of their relationships defines their identities.

What's more, some of the most frustrating and distressing experiences for people with ADHD are social interactions. Studies show that women with the condition have more impairment of social behaviors than women without the condition.

Emotional factors, such as fear and a mood disorder, weaken them. Friendships are about trust, knowledge of the needs of others, emotional support, and the preservation of relationships. These require an almost perfect choreography of executive functions, and women with ADHD often find themselves thwarted as they try to dance to the tune of friendship.

The myth is that it's easier for women to maintain relationships, and women with ADHD strive to hide their social impairments. We want friends and need them, but they're afraid they're being outed as a scam. Amber described the feeling like an impostor: "If they're not inviting me to join the book club, I'm a rejection— but if they invite me, they'll find out I hate reading." Friendships require verbal interplay, good listening, and awareness of nonverbal signs.

Many women with ADHD find it difficult to perform those skills consistently. Juggling complicated lives, many women have little energy left over to maintain close friendships. Their lives require a regrouping of downtimes. At night, when they don't have to be with anyone, they rejoice in the quiet moments. Now, seeking communication, they pledge too much to be welcomed in their endeavors.

Understanding the time, money, and preparation required, Jen confessed, "I've always made excuses to avoid breakfasts for preschool moms. And I decided to run the Auction when they asked me to volunteer. I thought I could feel less guilty and make them like me. I didn't consider myself ignorant about auctions. I certainly wouldn't ask them for help after volunteering, so I drove myself and my family crazy trying to score some credibility with the moms. "Most women with ADHD carry painful memories of friendships that have gone wrong, and fears of objection and rejection are increasing their avoidance.

As women with ADHD spend time with good friends, they can be fully present— optimistic and enthusiastic. But they can't retain the emotional memory when the mates are done. Moved by more urgent matters to the back burner, the mates slip off the radar screen so treasured they may be.

Unfortunately, women with ADHD may not note the growing alienation from their mates. Maintaining friendship demands that you check-in and say, "How are you?" Even if not much has happened since the friends had spoken last time. Cara fretted, "Did Amanda tell me that she had divorced her mother, or had a hip replacement? I'm not sure, but I know that she knows all I'm telling her.'

Friendship Shame for Women with ADHD

Social expectations include birthday cards, thank-you notes, and the like. Check-ins are often moved from the to-dodo list of today to the list of tomorrow until they are postponed for days, weeks, or months. Long silences do not mean a lack of interest, but that is how friends view them. Many women with ADHD become ashamed of their isolation after a contact break and afraid of its implications, so they let the relationship slip away rather than attempt to explain their silence.

A challenge lies in the reciprocal invitation. For example, Ashley has mentioned the lengths to which she goes when she has to reciprocate for a dinner. "I dump all the household junk into garbage bags the night before my dinner party and fire them into the closet where they're living for months. I refuse kitchen aid proposals so no one sees the crumbs in the refrigerator. Because I am so anxious, I can't enjoy my evenings. "Internalizing the shame may keep your missteps a secret, but it also keeps your authentic self-hidden.

Social Strategies for Women with ADHD

Your ADHD Brain Technology Harness Technology will improve social interaction. Friends want an acknowledgment, but they don't need to get it in the mail.

- A single-line text ("Thinking of you") breaks the silence and is valued.

- You can rely on pop-up alerts and alarms to help you recall important dates.

- Set the alarm to indicate the time when you need to leave for lunch, instead of the lunchtime itself, to avoid being late for a lunch date. Be patient in calculating travel time, so you don't get into a frenzy.

- You can have alarms empower you if you pay attention to them. "I'm going to do it in a minute" helps the brain to move on to something else. Eliminate using the "snooze" feature on alarms and attempt to commit just to stand up when the alarm goes off. Standing up does not allow for tenderness.

Talk Openly About Your ADHD Symptoms

Socialize with versatile mates, and embrace your ways. Some friends expect total and immediate attention, and consider any delay to be negligent. Without apology, you can explain your situation: "I'm not great to respond quickly, but I consider your emails important to me. I'll get back to you soon. "When sustaining a relationship causes more anxiety, remorse, and self-doubt than satisfaction, think of those costs while you analyze your friendship.

Anticipate Your ADHD Triggers

Keep your red flags in mind. People with ADHD don't feel as comfortable as team players. We tend to feel that their differences preclude party or group membership. As the ADHD brain continues to seek gratification, some may be prompted to disrupt conversations, change the subject, break eye contact, or tune it out. If you're gathering at a restaurant around a table, sit down near the center. For people on both sides, when you lose interest, you can choose the speaker who hires you and switch conversations. If you start fidgeting, stifling a yawn, or checking the time, appreciate the need to move on with your brain. Use the toilet — to refresh and to renew. Check your phone, walk around, and maybe come back with a reason to leave early.

Incorporate Movement into Your Plans

Replace a shopping day by a stroll or a lunch date. A lot of women enjoy shopping together but typically not women with ADHD. In a multi-sensory environment, they need to go at their own pace. In this environment, attending to the needs of another person is usually stressful, and leaves people with ADHD feeling trapped and irritated. Most say yes to a casual invitation to go shopping, but they want to go out when the date comes. It is better to say when you're making plans, "Shopping isn't my strong suit. How about instead going for a walk or lunch?"

How to Host a Dinner Party with ADHD?

Use these strategies when reciprocating a dinner date:

- If you can eat outside and have less formal buffet-style meals, try your hosting in warmer weather.

- For the same evening, several people are inviting everyone they owe dinner to get several responsibilities over at once. Sure, you just have to cook one meal, but there's too much focus on attending to everyone at once.

- You can create a distraction with a small group: play a game, share some new music that you've heard, or take a walk after dinner.

- Guide the discussion to topics you feel confident about. Try to keep short the evening, considering early on that the next day you need to get a jump. This offers structure by setting a boundary in place.

- Another option is to deliver an entirely different experience, which will reciprocate without the war. Take friends out for high tea, or have a picnic lunch prepared in the park.

Accept Your Brain

You cannot change your brain wiring or the world's standards. But you can comprehend that the truth we see is colored by the lens we see through. The good news is that the value of standards can be reframed so that they have less control over you. The goal is to see the world through a lens that embraces your unique needs. Relieved from social constraints and assumptions, instead of apologizing for your responsibilities, you will act on your strengths. Through learning to put your own ideals above the demands of the world, you will balance your needs against the needs of others. You will gain confidence, with respect for your struggles, to make and sustain the friendships that support you.

What's Your Friendship Type?

Women with ADHD, depending on their ADHD subtype, have specific obstacles to having and retaining mates. Those with ADHD that is hyperactive/impulsive:

· Interrupt discussions are easily bored

· Dominate discourse ignore social rules

· Blurt out negative comments

· Complain about themselves using too much alcohol to improve their level of stimulation

· Frequency relationships that feel stressful

Those with Inattentive ADHD:

· Feel overwhelmed by emotional

· Demands experience distress in new social situations

· Censoring themselves while perceiving conflict

· Avoiding unstructured group socializing

· Withdrawal while feeling over-stimulated

· Using obsessive habits to build a faultless

· Façade attributing their errors to character

· Defects expecting disapproval or rejection

Chapter 10: Improving Executive Functioning

Executive function is the cognitive process that organizes thoughts and events, prioritizes tasks, effectively controls time, and makes decisions. Executive function skills are the skills that enable us to develop project management frameworks and strategies and to decide the actions required to move through the project forward. Individuals with executive impairment often have difficulty evaluating, preparing, arranging, scheduling, and completing tasks at all — or on time. They misplace materials, prioritize things wrong, and are overwhelmed by large projects.

Was Executive Dysfunction An ADHD Symptom?

There's a lot of confusion about "executive function"— and how it's ADHD related. Was ADHD a behavioral disorder? Is ADHD also any executive function disorder? The responses depend on what "executive functions" we mean— and how they apply to self-regulation.

In the 1970s, Karl Pribram coined the term "executive functioning," whose work suggested that the executive functions were predominantly regulated by psychology and psychiatry. Nevertheless, it has expanded in recent years into the wider field of general psychology and education, where it is also integrated into teaching strategies and arrangements in the classroom.

So far, we are aware of four circuits in the brain's prefrontal cortex that relates to executive function— and executive dysfunction.

10.1: Executive Function and the ADHD Brain

-The What Circuit: Going back from the frontal lobe— particularly the outer surface — to an area of the brain called the basal ganglia, especially the structure called the striatum.

The "What "Circuit is connected to working memory, so what we think starts to direct what we do in this circuit. This is especially when it comes to plans, goals, and the future.

–The When Circuit: This second circuit goes back from the same prefrontal region to a very old part of the brain called the cerebellum, at the back of the head. The "When" Circuit is the brain's pacing circuit— it controls not only how smooth activity is going to be and the sequence of behavior but also the timeliness of your behaviors and when you do other things. An incorrectly functioning "When" Circuit in an ADHD person explains why we often have time management problems.

The "Why" circuit: The third circuit also originates from the front lobe, passing through the central part of the brain (known as the anterior cingulate) to tonsillitis — the gateway to the limbic system. It's often called the "hot" circuit because it's connected to our emotions— it's where we think how we feel influences it, and vice versa. In all our plans, it is the final decision-maker. This is the circuit that ultimately selects among the options based on how we feel about them and their emotional and motivational properties when thinking about multiple things we might be doing.

–The "Who" Circuit: This final circuit travels from the front lobe to the hemisphere's very center. It's where self-awareness occurs— it's where we're aware of what we're doing, how we feel (both internally and externally), and what's going on with us.

You can understand where the signs begin by presenting ADHD in relation to those four circuits. Depending on which circuits are most impaired and least impaired, you can see the difference in the types of symptoms each person will have. Some people have more deficits in working memory. Many people have problems with controlling emotions more. Many people have more problems with pacing, but all the others have fewer difficulties. But all of them involve those circuits.

10.2: What Are the Core Executive Function Skills?

Okay, we know what aspects of the executive brain control functions, but exactly what are they? Executive function broadly refers to the cognitive or mental abilities people need to pursue goals actively. In other words, it's about how we conduct ourselves towards our future goals and what mental abilities we need to achieve them.

The concept is closely related to self-regulation— executive roles are actions that you are doing to yourself to alter your behavior. You're hoping to change the life for the better by successfully using your executive functions.

The quality of those seven abilities is measured by the executive function:

1. Self-awareness: This is, to put it simply, self-directed attention.

2. Inhibition: Known also as self-restraint.

3. Non-Verbal Working Memory: Capability of keeping things in your mind. Visual imagery, in essence— how well you can visually visualize things.

4. Verbal working memory: speech of oneself or speech of one's own. Most people consider this to be their "inner monologue."

5. Emotional self-regulation: The ability to take on and use the four previous executive functions to manipulate your own emotional state. It means learning how to use words, pictures, and your own self-awareness to process and change our feelings about things.

6. Self-motivation: How well you can motivate yourself when there is no immediate external impact to accomplish a mission.

7. Planning and Problem Solving: Many experts like to think of this as "self-play"— how we play with knowledge in our minds and come up with new ways to do something. We're preparing solutions to our problems by taking things apart and recombining them in different ways.

Sounds familiar to that list? It ought to. Someone showing the typical ADHD signs will have difficulty with all or most of these seven executive functions. Inhibition issues in someone with ADHD result, for example, with impulsive actions. Emotional compliance issues lead to unacceptable outbursts.

ADHD is basically an Executive Deficit Development Disorder (EFDD). The paragliding term "ADHD" is simply another way to refer to those issues.

Those seven executive functions develop in generally chronological order over time. Self-awareness begins to develop around age 2, and the planning and problem-solving in a neurotypical person should be fully developed by age 30. Those with ADHD are usually around 30-40% behind their peers in switching from one executive function to another. Therefore, it makes sense for children and adults with ADHD to have trouble handling age-appropriate circumstances — they think and act in ways that are much like younger people.

10.3: Ways to improve executive function

ADHD is seen by many as a problem with focus, attention, and hyperactivity. However, recent research shows that deficits in executive function cause more impairment in the personal and professional lives of individuals. Executive function includes all the following cognitive skills: planning, prioritizing, strategizing, motivating, initiating tasks, organizing, performing complex tasks, and focusing on details; there is some controversy, however, overall the functions included in the executive functions class.

Executive function tends to be very less responsive to adult ADHD medications compared to the 70-80 percent high success rate for other core ADHD symptoms such as focus, hyperactivity, attention, impulsivity, and distractibility. Adults with ADHD thus continue to experience challenges in the workplace and in their personal lives.

Understanding and addressing executive-function challenges is essential in helping adults with ADHD address this condition in full.

Take Winnie*, for example, who is a 28-year-old woman who finished business school last year and is currently working in accounting for a real estate firm. Due to careless mistakes, missed deadlines, and poor results, her boss was very dissatisfied with her performance. She is on a probationary period of two months and is panicking. She has, therefore, contacted me to address her insomnia, anxiety, and whether her past diagnosis of ADHD currently affects her career.

Winnie was diagnosed with ADHD, a type of hyperactivity when she was in fourth grade, and she had several years of help with medications. She was also fortunate to receive comprehensive tutoring in all of her subjects, and she performed well in school. As she moved to another state, though, her parents decided not to continue therapy. She carried her tutoring going.

She struggled with high school and college, with focus, attention, and time management challenges. She worked in sales for several years after college and did very well. She loved entertaining customers and was very productive except with her work's boring aspects such as expense reports and monthly reports. She sometimes worked on a project for weeks and then, when she met her boss, she found that she had underestimated the project's intent and focus, and had to start from scratch. She was constantly depressed, overwhelmed, and felt behind. She didn't know each day which project or task was beginning and would often switch from task to task or stop doing her job altogether.

I conducted a thorough psychiatric evaluation of her history and current symptoms at the time we met. I demonstrated to her that she was suffering from ADHD and that these symptoms sometimes persist into adult life. I have clarified to her that trouble with executive functioning is the significant challenge of ADHD. It was evident from her experience that her anxiety and insomnia were secondary to her on-office challenges.

I restarted her on Adderall as well as a centered Cognitive Behavioral Therapy course to teach her cognitive skills, behavioral approaches, and emotional control methods to overcome the problems of her executive functions. Efficiency and productivity had dramatically improved within four weeks. She had a follow-up meeting with her boss, who was quite impressed with their new performance standard. She got promoted to a higher-level position within a year.

For those dealing with executive function deficits like Winnie, here are five techniques that can improve performance and efficiency, especially within the workplace.

Clarify Expectations.

People with ADHD are mostly very creative and full of energy. As one of my mentors is known for saying, people with ADHD are like fast race cars without brakes working, they jump with excitement out of doors, but not usually with practical or well-thought-out objectives. Unlike Winnie, several people will work for weeks but fail to reach the goals the team is looking for. So always clarify your expectations with your customer, boss, or manager. Here are a few questions you maybe want to ask: How does this particular project look like success? What is Project Timeframe? What is that project's scope? Are we aiming for broad strokes and concepts or for drilling down to the details of granules?

Request Feedback.

Those with ADHD have often also struggled with many defeats or disappointments in their lives. They are thus burdened with substantial self-doubt and embarrassment and stop checking in with the team or boss or seeking input, fearing exposure to possible criticism.

 Besides clarifying expectations, it is important that you get feedback about your work throughout the project, particularly early in the process. One individual with whom I worked avoided asking for any input on a large project and found after three months that he had interesting ideas, but these ideas were in conflict with the vision of the team leader.

As part of the business policy, Winnie generally met with her boss on a monthly basis. Nonetheless, I suggested that she also meet with her boss twice a week for ten minutes to make sure that her growth and quality of work meets standards. Winnie said these two-week meetings have helped her with transparency and strengthened her level of motivation and trust. Her manager also commented on the dedication of Winnie and its newfound commitment.

Hand Writes a Strategy.

Winnie and a lot of my patients are undertaking big projects without a written strategy. This is like sailing a boat to Europe without a map or a compass. Others might avoid taking on the projects involved because they are overwhelmed by the idea.

Take out a sheet of paper or notebook and write down the specific steps for the project before you even embark on any project, large or small. And, I want to emphasize the part about handwriting it out. People suffering from ADHD are often visual and kinesthetic learners. Writing out the plan by hand instead of typing it on a keyboard will dramatically improve your skill and imagination in planning. It doesn't have to be written exactly and can be a fluid, roundabout operation. You may not even expect all of the initial steps. In that scenario, one of the steps might be to pose a certain question to a trusted adviser or to do some analysis. Some of the steps may be too detailed and may need to be broken down into smaller steps, especially if they are nebulous or seem daunting.

Winnie arrived at our session frenzied about an imminent presentation to a senior vice-president of the company during one of our initial meetings. Together we developed a handwritten, step-by-step presentation strategy. She was not only calmer by the end of our session but also enthusiastic about getting started. A few sessions later, she reported that her presentation received a stellar reception.

Maintain a Coordinated Task list and Calendar.

I've got a saying to my patients:' if it's not on the calendar, it doesn't exist.' What this means is that if a job or the to-dodo item is not entered or reported on a specific time period on the calendar, there's a good chance that it will be missed or' cracked down.'

Once all of the steps in the project have been listed, write every step in your calendar at a particular date and time. They may not be aware of the specific times an object will actually be done, or when a higher priority task may be involved. But making an informed guess about the potential times when a task is likely to be worked on enhances your chances of success as well as helps you feel calmer and less overwhelmed moving forward. Moreover, having a written schedule that displays all your activities in one place helps you plan and focus on the job you are doing.

You should also put other activities, meetings, social or networking events, lectures, and appointments on your calendar. I consider using a "week-at-a-glance" planner to have a summary of the whole week showing how the various roles and activities interact and interconnect. Personally, I prefer an old-fashioned paper calendar, since people with ADHD still work better with handwriting than using a digital calendar on the screen.

Likewise, I recommend having a notebook to use as your task notebook, such as a hardcover Moleskin. You can write down all of your to - do's in one position here and avoid the issue of having items written in multiple locations. Each notebook page represents a separate day and includes all of the tasks, phone calls, and notes that occur on that day. Once again, every task in the calendar should also be written at a specific time.

Create Your Master Handbook.

Individuals with Adult ADHD are often unaware of a company's or team's "rules." Such pieces of information may include the company-specific parameters of documents or presentations, the arrangement of files, and regulations for compliance. It may also contain passwords, protocols, and standards of unwritten use.

One of my patients was expected to arrange a quarterly meeting that included all the top-level managers with very clear invitation criteria, scheduling a conference room in advance, asking for guest speakers, and a huge amount of small but important information. He would always get really anxious because, after the quarterly meeting, he would generally forget many of the specifics of this process. We wrote down the specific pieces of information in his own "Master Manual" to support him. Therefore, he had all the information at his disposal every fifth and then felt calmer and in control of the situation.

Summary.

Executive functioning deficiencies are a major stumbling block and obstacle for individuals with Adult ADHD. Using these management approaches and techniques will greatly help enhance executive functioning and achieve the progress you're striving for in your personal and professional lives.

Winnie continued improving over the following months of treatment. Originally, we met every two weeks to discuss strategies and competencies. However, when Winnie continued to incorporate the new habits, we didn't have to meet as often and are meeting every month or two at best. She has made tremendous progress over the past year and was elevated to team leader a second time. She manages a team of four and remains very well focused on her assignments, priorities, and the success of the whole team. Although some tasks fall by the wayside, and she does not always adhere perfectly to the strategies, she has come a long way to becoming a valued leader and an integral part of the firm.

By using these techniques, many of my patients have greatly increased their professional and personal performance, and being a part of this journey has been extremely rewarding. Some of those strategies might not apply in exactly the same way to you or your work. However, when individuals with adult ADHD implement these approaches and fine-tune them to match their individual needs, significant gains can often occur.

Chapter 11: Success habits

Any adult with ADHD has special talents. The trick is to discover them — and use them to attain important objectives. Know how to get coordinated, and how to know how to delegate.

1. Do what you're good at.

Everyone is good at certain things, not so good at others. Focusing on strengthening your strengths is often more successful, rather than trying to shore up your weak points. So, when you have to do something that you're not especially good at? Consult with members of your family, mentors or tutors to find coping strategies that will help you become "strong enough."

2. Keep in touch with your friends.

Good friends are key to happiness. And friends will give you a valuable perspective.

3. Ask for advice.

Life is tricky but you don't have to go it alone. Figure who you trust, and regularly confer with them – and especially when issues arise. Ignore finger-wagers and the naysayers.

4. Get enough organized.

You don't have to organize yourself absolutely — perfect files, no clutter. For most, that's too hard, and to my mind, nothing but a waste of your time. You just need to be disciplined enough to keep the disorganization from getting in your way.

5. Find an outlet for your creativity.

What are your hobbies? Music?-Music? Karate-Karate? I write my outlet. When I'm engaged in a writing project, life is always more exciting and satisfying.

6. Learn to delegate.

If you're faced with a specific difficult task or obligation, ask someone else to do it for you in return for doing something for him. And don't think that when you don't get things done someone else will pick up the slack for you. Tell him or her to do just that. In the context of marriage, asking for help is particularly important; failing to acknowledge that you are leaving the not - so-fun stuff (housekeeping, bill-paying, etc.) to a partner without ADHD invariably leads to resentments.

7. Stay optimistic.

Everyone has a dark side, and sometimes they may feel down. But do your best with your optimistic side to make choices and to "run your life."

Conclusion:

Disorder of attention deficit hyperactivity (ADHD) affects children and adolescents, which can extend into adulthood. The most frequently diagnosed developmental mental disorder is ADHD. Kids with ADHD are inherently hyperactive and unable to control their impulses. And, they may have trouble paying attention.

Condition of attention deficit hyperactivity (ADHD) is a type of neurodevelopmental mental disorder. It is defined by difficulties in paying attention, repetitive behavior and behaving without regard to consequences, which otherwise are not appropriate for a person's age. Individuals with ADHD may also exhibit anger control problems. The signs should begin before a person is twelve years of age for a diagnosis, be present for more than six months, and cause problems in at least two environments (such as school, home, or recreation).

Problems with paying attention in children may result in poor performance at the school. There is also a correlation with other mental disorders and abuse of the drugs. Although it causes disability, especially in modern society, many people with ADHD may tend to be concerned with tasks they find interesting or satisfying (known as hyper focus).

Neurodiversity is a concept which, like any other human variation, recognizes and acknowledges the neurological variations. These variants may include Dyspraxia, Dyslexia, Dyscalculia, Attention Deficit Hyperactivity Disorder, and Autistic Spectrum related variations. Figures across the industry will range from 10-20 per cent.

Understand how our brains work, most of us have variations in our tolerance and response to noise, stimulation, social activity and how much information we can easily consume before our minds feel overwhelmed and depleted. To adapt to the occupations or circumstances, we may need to use techniques.

It is very important for us to embrace neurodiversity and accept the neurodiverse people as normal we should recognize the level and area of their intelligence and let them grow in that field so they could have normal and easy life which they could enjoy.

We should be planned and given to learning products and techniques according to their abilities and talents so that they can improve their skills and have a successful career in them.

Neurodiverse must also realize their positions and should start working smartly so that they can play a vital role in society and fulfill their duties and live life with respect and achievement to the fullest.

The women have a significant and powerful role in our society, as she has many hundreds of duties to perform and obstacles to tackle while suffering from ADHD, making it harder for her to get things done.

In that situation, she has to tolerate her differences, and she has to manage things smartly and get balanced enough to maintain her home with her family and work at the same time, instead of getting tired or broken. She can use smart tactics, methods, and technology to quickly and efficiently get her tasks done on time.

Reference:

Adult attention-deficit/hyperactivity disorder (ADHD) - Symptoms and causes. Retrieved from **https://www.mayoclinic.org/diseases-conditions/adult-adhd/symptoms-causes/syc-20350878**

Why Many Women with ADHD Remain Undiagnosed? Retrieved from **https://www.verywellmind.com/add-symptoms-in-women-20394**

What is ADHD? Retrieved from **https://www.cdc.gov/ncbddd/adhd/facts.html**

Succeeding in the Workplace - CHADD. Retrieved from **https://chadd.org/for-adults/succeeding-in-the-workplace/**

How to Make Friends as an Adult Woman With ADHD. Retrieved from **https://www.additudemag.com/how-to-make-friends-adult-woman/**

The Effects of ADHD on Communication. Retrieved from **https://www.addrc.org/effects-adhd-communication/**

Segal, R Tips for Managing Adult ADHD. Retrieved from **https://www.helpguide.org/articles/add-adhd/managing-adult-adhd-attention-deficit-disorder.htm**

CPSIA information can be obtained
at www.ICGtesting.com
Printed in the USA
LVHW080059230221
679685LV00017B/2751